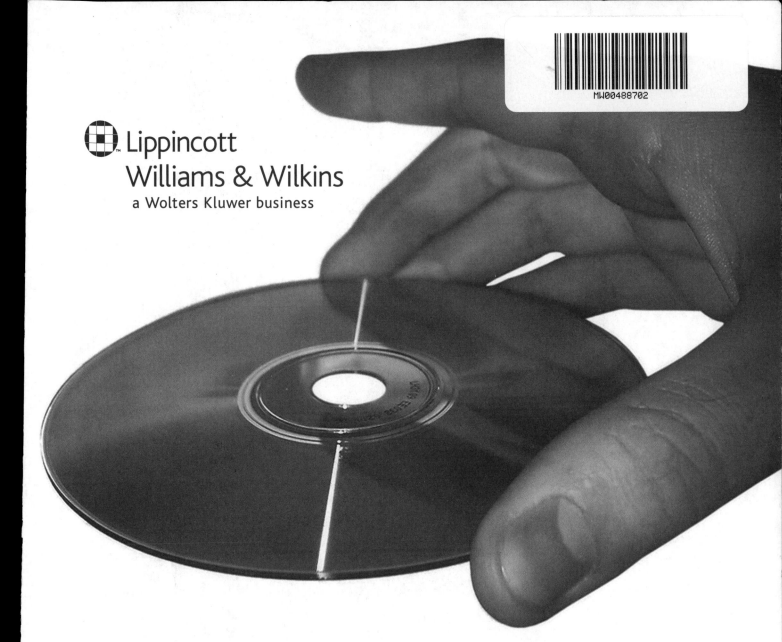

**Lippincott
Williams & Wilkins**
a Wolters Kluwer business

# CD Included!

*Look inside for your
300-question pretest and
300-question posttest!*

# PANCE/PANRE Flash Review

# PANCE/PANRE Flash Review

Debbie Winberry, PA-C

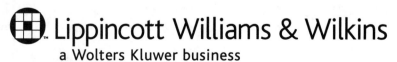 Lippincott Williams & Wilkins
a Wolters Kluwer business

Philadelphia · Baltimore · New York · London
Buenos Aires · Hong Kong · Sydney · Tokyo

*Acquisitions Editor:* Nancy Anastasi Duffy
*Managing Editor:* Kathleen H. Scogna
*Marketing Manager:* Emilie Linkins
*Production Editor:* Sirkka E. H. Bertling
*Design Coordinator:* Holly Reid McLaughlin
*Interior Designer:* Mary McKeon
*Cover Designer:* Christine Jenny
*Compositor:* Circle Graphics, Inc.
*Printer:* Data Reproductions Corporation

**Library of Congress Cataloging-in-Publication Data**

Winberry, Debbie.
  PANCE/PANRE flash review / Debbie Winberry.
    p. ; cm.
  ISBN-13: 978-1-4051-0508-8
  ISBN-10: 1-4051-0508-9
  1. Physicians' assistants—Examinations, questions, etc. I. Title.
  [DNLM: 1. Physician Assistants—Examination Questions. 2. Certification—Examination Questions. W 18.2 W758p 2007]
  R697.P45W56 2007
  610.73'72076—dc22

                                                                              2006004931

To Stephen and my parents

# PREFACE

The goal of this book is to help the physician assistant pass the NCCPA (National Commission on Certification of Physician Assistants) recertification exam. My goal was to make reviewing for the Physician Assistant National Recertification Examination (PANRE) as easy and painless as possible. This book was written primarily for those PAs who have been practicing in a specialty area and are concerned about preparing for another primary care exam. The goals of PAs who have been specializing for the past 5 or more years are not always the same as those of seasoned primary care PAs. That said, however, this book can be used by any PA. It does not presuppose a specific level of knowledge in any one area but reviews all the basic concepts. After using this book, you should be able to feel confident in sitting for the PANRE no matter how much (or how little) you may have retained since your last NCCPA exam.

The materials in this book and on the accompanying CD were designed to match the content, complexity, and type of questions seen on the PANCE and PANRE exams. The allotment of questions for both the pre- and posttests approximates the NCCPA's published blueprint for content for the exams. The book and CD are divided into three distinct sections:

1. A 300-question pretest on the CD to determine your preparedness before your review begins. This will allow you to determine your areas of weakness. Refer to page xi for information about the NCCPA's percentage of each area on the exam.
2. A review section, which is set up in flash card style for easy review of important information on specific diseases and disorders.
3. A 300-question posttest on the CD to determine your readiness for the exam.

Because of the large amount of information presented in a condensed space, you will find many abbreviations used throughout the book. I have tried to use the most widely known of these, but some may not be familiar to everyone. You will find an exhaustive list of all the abbreviations used listed in alphabetical order in Appendix 1, which will help you to identify those you do not recognize. I have also used the common names for specific "syndromes" or signs that are universally recognized, such as "Roth's spots" or "Homans' sign." You will find descriptions of these in Appendix 2, "Terminology Links."

This book will help to prepare you for either the PANCE or PANRE exam. I further believe that it will become an important review book to be used by any practicing PA in his or her clinical practice.

# ACKNOWLEDGMENT

This book marks the culmination of a path the Lord set me on years ago when I took my first medical course at a junior college in California. I would like to acknowledge Mr. Steven Williams, the instructor I had for my first EMT course, who told me to "continue on in medicine." Steve, you will never know how those simple words affected me.

# NCCPA Blueprint for PANCE/PANRE Examinations

Two dimensions are tested on the PANCE/PANRE examinations:

1. Organ systems and the diseases, disorders, and medical assessments physician assistants encounter within those systems

2. The knowledge and skills physician assistants should exhibit when confronted with those diseases, disorders, and assessments

Also, at least 20% of the questions will be related to surgery, and up to 2% will be legal or ethical questions.

| Percent of Exam Content | Diseases, Disorders, & Medical Assessments | Percent of Exam Content | Knowledge & Skill Areas |
|---|---|---|---|
| 16 | Cardiovascular System | 16 | Hx Taking & Performing PE |
| 12 | Pulmonary System | 14 | Using Lab & Dx Studies |
| 10 | Gastrointestinal System/Nutrition | 18 | Formulating Most Likely Dx |
| 10 | Musculoskeletal System | 14 | Clinical Intervention |
| 9 | EENT | 18 | Clinical Therapeutics |
| 8 | Reproductive System | 10 | Health Maintenance |
| 6 | Endocrine System | 10 | Applying Scientific Concepts |
| 6 | Neurologic System | | |
| 6 | Psychiatry/Behavioral Science | 100% | |
| 6 | Genitourinary System | | |
| 5 | Dermatologic System | | |
| 3 | Hematologic System | | |
| 3 | Infectious Diseases | | |
| 100% | | | |

# CONTENTS

*Preface* . . . . . . . . . . . . . . . . . . . . . . . . . . . . . . . . . . . . . . . . . . . . . . . . . . . . . . . . . . . . . . . . . . . *vii*

*Acknowledgment* . . . . . . . . . . . . . . . . . . . . . . . . . . . . . . . . . . . . . . . . . . . . . . . . . . . . . . . . . . . . . *ix*

*NCCPA Blueprint for PANCE/PANRE Examinations* . . . . . . . . . . . . . . . . . . . . . . . . . . . . . . . . *xi*

**Cardiovascular System** . . . . . . . . . . . . . . . . . . . . . . . . . . . . . . . . . . . . . . . . . . . . . . . . . . . . . . .1

    Card 1.1  Angina Pectoris . . . . . . . . . . . . . . . . . . . . . . . . . . . . . . . . . . . . . . . . . . . . . . . . .2

    Card 1.2  Angina Pectoris, Specific Types . . . . . . . . . . . . . . . . . . . . . . . . . . . . . . . . . . . .2

    Card 1.3  Aortic Aneurysm . . . . . . . . . . . . . . . . . . . . . . . . . . . . . . . . . . . . . . . . . . . . . . . .3

    Card 1.4  Atrioventricular (AV) Heart Blocks . . . . . . . . . . . . . . . . . . . . . . . . . . . . . . . . .3

    Card 1.5  Bacterial Endocarditis . . . . . . . . . . . . . . . . . . . . . . . . . . . . . . . . . . . . . . . . . . .4

    Card 1.6  Bacterial Endocarditis: Duke Diagnostic Criteria . . . . . . . . . . . . . . . . . . . . .4

    Card 1.7  Buerger's Disease (Thromboangiitis Obliterans) . . . . . . . . . . . . . . . . . . . . .5

    Card 1.8  Cardiogenic Shock . . . . . . . . . . . . . . . . . . . . . . . . . . . . . . . . . . . . . . . . . . . . .5

    Card 1.9A  Cardiomyopathy . . . . . . . . . . . . . . . . . . . . . . . . . . . . . . . . . . . . . . . . . . . . .6

    Card 1.9B  Cardiomyopathy, Continued . . . . . . . . . . . . . . . . . . . . . . . . . . . . . . . . . . . .6

    Card 1.10  Congenital Heart Defects: Atrial Septal Defect . . . . . . . . . . . . . . . . . . . . .7

    Card 1.11  Congenital Heart Defects: Coarctation of the Aorta . . . . . . . . . . . . . . . . .7

    Card 1.12  Congenital Heart Defects: Patent Ductus Arteriosus . . . . . . . . . . . . . . . . .8

    Card 1.13  Congenital Heart Defects: Pulmonary Stenosis . . . . . . . . . . . . . . . . . . . . .8

    Card 1.14  Congenital Heart Defects: Tetralogy of Fallot . . . . . . . . . . . . . . . . . . . . . .9

    Card 1.15  Congenital Heart Defects: Ventricular Septal Defect . . . . . . . . . . . . . . . . .9

    Card 1.16A  Congestive Heart Failure . . . . . . . . . . . . . . . . . . . . . . . . . . . . . . . . . . . .10

    Card 1.16B  Congestive Heart Failure, Continued . . . . . . . . . . . . . . . . . . . . . . . . . . .10

    Card 1.17  Coronary Artery Disease . . . . . . . . . . . . . . . . . . . . . . . . . . . . . . . . . . . . . .11

    Card 1.18  Deep Venous Thrombosis . . . . . . . . . . . . . . . . . . . . . . . . . . . . . . . . . . . . .11

    Card 1.19  Dysrhythmias: Bradydysrhythmias . . . . . . . . . . . . . . . . . . . . . . . . . . . . . .12

    Card 1.20  Dysrhythmias: Bradydysrhythmias, Specific Types . . . . . . . . . . . . . . . . .12

    Card 1.21  Dysrhythmias: Tachydysrhythmias . . . . . . . . . . . . . . . . . . . . . . . . . . . . . .13

    Card 1.22A  Dysrhythmias: Tachydysrhythmias, Specific Types . . . . . . . . . . . . . . . .14

    Card 1.22B  Dysrhythmias: Tachydysrhythmias, Specific Types, Continued . . . . . . .14

    Card 1.23A  ECG Essentials . . . . . . . . . . . . . . . . . . . . . . . . . . . . . . . . . . . . . . . . . . . .15

    Card 1.23B  ECG Essentials, Continued . . . . . . . . . . . . . . . . . . . . . . . . . . . . . . . . . . .15

    Card 1.24  Heart Sounds . . . . . . . . . . . . . . . . . . . . . . . . . . . . . . . . . . . . . . . . . . . . . .16

    Card 1.25  Hypertension . . . . . . . . . . . . . . . . . . . . . . . . . . . . . . . . . . . . . . . . . . . . . .16

    Card 1.26  Hypertension, Specific Types . . . . . . . . . . . . . . . . . . . . . . . . . . . . . . . . . .17

    Card 1.27A  Murmurs . . . . . . . . . . . . . . . . . . . . . . . . . . . . . . . . . . . . . . . . . . . . . . . .17

    Card 1.27B  Murmurs, Continued . . . . . . . . . . . . . . . . . . . . . . . . . . . . . . . . . . . . . . .18

    Card 1.28  Myocardial Infarction . . . . . . . . . . . . . . . . . . . . . . . . . . . . . . . . . . . . . . .18

    Card 1.29  Myocarditis . . . . . . . . . . . . . . . . . . . . . . . . . . . . . . . . . . . . . . . . . . . . . . .19

    Card 1.30  Pericardial Disorders . . . . . . . . . . . . . . . . . . . . . . . . . . . . . . . . . . . . . . . .19

Card 1.31  Pericarditis ......................................................20

Card 1.32  Peripheral Vascular Disease ...................................20

Card 1.33  Peripheral Vascular Disease: Fontaine Diagnostic Classification .......21

Card 1.34  Rheumatic Heart Disease .......................................21

Card 1.35  Rheumatic Heart Disease: Duckett-Jones Diagnostic Criteria .........22

Card 1.36  Sudden Cardiac Death ...........................................22

Card 1.37  Valvular Diseases: Aortic Regurgitation ........................23

Card 1.38  Valvular Diseases: Aortic Stenosis ............................23

Card 1.39  Valvular Diseases: Mitral Regurgitation .......................24

Card 1.40  Valvular Diseases: Mitral Stenosis ............................24

Card 1.41  Valvular Diseases: Mitral Valve Prolapse ......................25

Card 1.42  Valvular Diseases: Tricuspid Regurgitation ....................25

Card 1.43  Valvular Diseases: Tricuspid Stenosis .........................26

## Pulmonary System ...............................................................27

Card 2.1  Adult Respiratory Distress Syndrome ............................28

Card 2.2  Asbestos Pneumoconiosis .......................................28

Card 2.3  Asthma .........................................................29

Card 2.4  Asthma, Specific Types ........................................29

Card 2.5  Bronchiectasis ................................................30

Card 2.6  Bronchiolitis .................................................30

Card 2.7  Bronchitis, Acute ............................................31

Card 2.8  Bronchitis, Chronic (Type B COPD) ............................31

Card 2.9  Bronchogenic Carcinoma .......................................32

Card 2.10  Cystic Fibrosis ..............................................32

Card 2.11  Emphysema (Type A COPD) ......................................33

Card 2.12  Epiglottitis .................................................33

Card 2.13  Obstructive Sleep Apnea ......................................34

Card 2.14  Pleurisy .....................................................34

Card 2.15  Pneumonia ....................................................35

Card 2.16  Pneumonia, Specific Types ....................................35

Card 2.17  Pneumothorax .................................................36

Card 2.18  Pulmonary Embolism ...........................................36

Card 2.19  Pulmonary Tuberculosis .......................................37

Card 2.20  Sarcoidosis ..................................................37

Card 2.21  Solitary Pulmonary Nodule ....................................38

## Gastrointestinal System and Nutrition .........................................39

Card 3.1  Achalasia: Medical Perspective ................................40

Card 3.2  Acute Abdomen .................................................40

Card 3.3  Alcoholic Liver Disease .......................................41

Card 3.4  Anal Fissure ..................................................41

Card 3.5  Bowel Obstruction .............................................42

Card 3.6  Cirrhosis .....................................................42

Card 3.7  Cirrhosis, Primary Biliary ....................................43

Card 3.8  Colon Carcinoma ...............................................43

Card 3.9  Crohn's Disease ...............................................44

Card 3.10  Diverticular Disease .........................................44

Card 3.11  Esophageal Carcinoma ...............................................45

Card 3.12  Esophageal Varices .................................................45

Card 3.13  Esophagitis .......................................................46

Card 3.14  Gastric Carcinoma .................................................46

Card 3.15  Gastritis .........................................................47

Card 3.16  Gastroesophageal Reflux Disease ....................................47

Card 3.17  Hemochromatosis ..................................................48

Card 3.18  Hepatitis, Acute ...................................................48

Card 3.19  Hepatitis, Chronic .................................................49

Card 3.20A  Hepatitis, Specific Types ...........................................49

Card 3.20B  Hepatitis, Specific Types, Continued .................................50

Card 3.21  Hepatocellular Carcinoma ...........................................50

Card 3.22  Hiatal Hernia .....................................................51

Card 3.23  Hypertrophic Pyloric Stenosis .......................................51

Card 3.24  Intussusception ...................................................52

Card 3.25  Irritable Bowel Syndrome ...........................................52

Card 3.26  Jaundice of Infancy ................................................53

Card 3.27  Liver Abscess .....................................................53

Card 3.28  Malabsorption Syndromes ...........................................54

Card 3.29  Mallory-Weiss Syndrome ...........................................54

Card 3.30  Obesity ..........................................................55

Card 3.31  Pancreatic Carcinoma ..............................................55

Card 3.32  Pancreatitis, Chronic ..............................................56

Card 3.33  Peptic Ulcer Disease ...............................................56

Card 3.34  Sclerosing Cholangitis, Primary ......................................57

Card 3.35  Scurvy ...........................................................57

Card 3.36  Toxic Megacolon ..................................................58

Card 3.37  Ulcerative Colitis ..................................................58

**Musculoskeletal System** .......................................................**59**

Card 4.1  Adhesive Capsulitis .................................................60

Card 4.2  Ankle Fracture .....................................................60

Card 4.3  Ankle Sprain ......................................................61

Card 4.4  Ankylosing Spondylitis ..............................................61

Card 4.5  Anterior Cruciate Ligament (ACL) Injury ...............................62

Card 4.6  Avascular Necrosis ..................................................62

Card 4.7  Blount's Disease ....................................................63

Card 4.8  Carpal Tunnel Syndrome .............................................63

Card 4.9  Clubfoot Deformity .................................................64

Card 4.10  Colles' Fracture ...................................................64

Card 4.11  Cubital Tunnel Syndrome ...........................................65

Card 4.12  de Quervain's Tenosynovitis .........................................65

Card 4.13  Dysplasia of the Hip, Developmental ..................................66

Card 4.14  Epicondylitis, Lateral ..............................................66

Card 4.15  Epicondylitis, Medial ...............................................67

Card 4.16  Fibromyalgia ......................................................67

Card 4.17  Ganglion Cyst .....................................................68

Card 4.18  Gout ...........................................................................68

Card 4.19  Hand Infections: Felon ..................................................69

Card 4.20  Hand Infections: Flexor Tenosynovitis ..........................69

Card 4.21  Herniated Nucleus Pulposus ........................................70

Card 4.22  Legg-Calvé-Perthes Disease .........................................70

Card 4.23A  Low Back Pain ...........................................................71

Card 4.23B  Low Back Pain, Continued ..........................................71

Card 4.24  Mallet Finger ...............................................................72

Card 4.25  Medial Collateral Ligament Injuries ..............................72

Card 4.26  Meniscal Injury ............................................................73

Card 4.27  Metastatic Disease to Bone .........................................73

Card 4.28  Morton's Neuroma ......................................................74

Card 4.29  Nursemaid's Elbow .....................................................74

Card 4.30  Osteoarthritis ..............................................................75

Card 4.31  Paget's Disease ...........................................................75

Card 4.32  Rheumatoid Arthritis ...................................................76

Card 4.33  Rheumatoid Arthritis: Diagnostic Criteria .....................76

Card 4.34  Rotator Cuff Diseases ..................................................77

Card 4.35  Scoliosis ......................................................................77

Card 4.36  Shoulder Dislocation, Anterior ....................................78

Card 4.37  Shoulder Dislocation, Posterior ...................................78

Card 4.38  Slipped Capital Femoral Epiphysis ...............................79

Card 4.39  Spinal Stenosis ............................................................79

Card 4.40  Spondyloarthropathies ................................................80

Card 4.41  Systemic Lupus Erythematosus ....................................80

Card 4.42  Systemic Lupus Erythematosus: Diagnostic Criteria ......81

Card 4.43  Volkmann's Ischemic Contracture ................................81

**Eyes, Ears, Nose, and Throat** .......................................................82

Card 5.1  Acoustic Neuroma ........................................................83

Card 5.2  Amblyopia ....................................................................83

Card 5.3  Aphthous Stomatitis .....................................................84

Card 5.4  Cataracts ......................................................................84

Card 5.5  Central Retinal Artery Occlusion ...................................85

Card 5.6  Cholesteatoma .............................................................85

Card 5.7  Conjunctivitis ...............................................................86

Card 5.8  Epiglottitis ....................................................................86

Card 5.9  Epistaxis .......................................................................87

Card 5.10A  Eye Trauma: Abrasions ..............................................87

Card 5.10B  Eye Trauma: Burns ....................................................88

Card 5.10C  Eye Trauma: Foreign Bodies .......................................88

Card 5.10D  Eye Trauma: Lacerations ............................................89

Card 5.11  Glaucoma, Acute Angle Closure ...................................89

Card 5.12  Glaucoma, Primary Open Angle ...................................90

Card 5.13  Hearing Loss ...............................................................90

Card 5.14  Keith-Wagner-Barker Classification: Retinal Findings .....91

Card 5.15  Macular Degeneration .................................................91

Card 5.16  Optic Neuritis ..............................................................92

Card 5.17  Oral Candidiasis .......................................................92

Card 5.18  Otitis Externa .........................................................93

Card 5.19  Otitis Media, Acute ...................................................93

Card 5.20  Peritonsillar Abscess ..................................................94

Card 5.21  Retinal Detachment ...................................................94

Card 5.22  Rhinitis ...............................................................95

Card 5.23  Sinusitis ..............................................................95

Card 5.24  Vertigo ...............................................................96

**Reproductive System** ............................................................**97**

Card 6.1  Abruptio Placentae .....................................................98

Card 6.2  Adenomyosis ..........................................................98

Card 6.3  Benign Prostatic Hypertrophy ..........................................99

Card 6.4  Breast Carcinoma ......................................................99

Card 6.5  Cervical Carcinoma ....................................................100

Card 6.6  Cervical Carcinoma: Staging ...........................................100

Card 6.7  Ectopic Pregnancy .....................................................101

Card 6.8  Endometriosis .........................................................101

Card 6.9  Erectile Dysfunction ...................................................102

Card 6.10  Hormone Replacement Therapy ........................................102

Card 6.11  Hydatidiform Mole ....................................................103

Card 6.12  Mastitis ..............................................................103

Card 6.13  Menopause ...........................................................104

Card 6.14  Menstrual Cycle Phases ...............................................104

Card 6.15  Newborn Evaluation ..................................................105

Card 6.16  Oral Contraception Methods ...........................................105

Card 6.17  Ovarian Cysts and Tumors .............................................106

Card 6.18  Pelvic Inflammatory Disease ...........................................106

Card 6.19  Placenta Previa .......................................................107

Card 6.20  Polycystic Ovarian Syndrome ..........................................107

Card 6.21  Postpartum Hemorrhage ..............................................108

Card 6.22  Preeclampsia .........................................................108

Card 6.23  Pregnancy, Normal Signs ..............................................109

Card 6.24  Prenatal Care .........................................................109

Card 6.25  Prostate Carcinoma ...................................................110

Card 6.26  Prostatitis ............................................................110

Card 6.27A  Sexually Transmitted Diseases ........................................111

Card 6.27B  Sexually Transmitted Diseases, Continued .............................111

Card 6.28  Testicular Carcinoma ..................................................112

Card 6.29  Uterine Bleeding, Dysfunctional ........................................112

Card 6.30  Uterine Carcinoma ....................................................113

Card 6.31  Uterine Carcinoma: Staging for Endometrial Carcinoma .................113

Card 6.32  Uterine Leiomyoma (Fibroid) ..........................................114

Card 6.33  Vaginal Bleeding, Abnormal ...........................................114

**Endocrine System** ..............................................................**115**

Card 7.1  Acromegaly ...........................................................116

Card 7.2  Addison's Disease ......................................................116

Card 7.3    Adrenal Crisis ...................................................117

Card 7.4    Adrenal Hyperplasia, Congenital ...............................117

Card 7.5    Cushing's Syndrome ............................................118

Card 7.6    Diabetes Insipidus .............................................118

Card 7.7    Diabetes Mellitus ..............................................119

Card 7.8    Diabetic Ketoacidosis ..........................................119

Card 7.9    Graves' Disease ................................................120

Card 7.10   Hyperaldosteronism ............................................120

Card 7.11   Hyperparathyroidism ...........................................121

Card 7.12   Hyperpituitarism ..............................................121

Card 7.13   Hypopituitarism ...............................................122

Card 7.14   Hyperthyroidism ...............................................122

Card 7.15   Hypothyroidism ................................................123

Card 7.16   Klinefelter's Syndrome .........................................123

Card 7.17   Osteoporosis ..................................................124

Card 7.18   Pheochromocytoma .............................................124

Card 7.19   Syndrome of Inappropriate Antidiuretic Hormone (SIADH) .........125

Card 7.20   Thyroid Carcinoma .............................................125

Card 7.21   Thyroiditis ...................................................126

Card 7.22   Turner's Syndrome .............................................126

## Neurologic System ...............................................**127**

Card 8.1    Alzheimer's Disease ............................................128

Card 8.2    Amyotrophic Lateral Sclerosis ..................................128

Card 8.3    Bell's Palsy ..................................................129

Card 8.4    Cerebrovascular Accident .......................................129

Card 8.5    Cranial Nerves ................................................130

Card 8.6    Dementia and Delirium, Comparison .............................130

Card 8.7    Encephalitis ..................................................131

Card 8.8    Guillain-Barré Syndrome ........................................131

Card 8.9    Headache .....................................................132

Card 8.10   Huntington's Chorea ...........................................132

Card 8.11   Hydrocephalus, Normal Pressure ................................133

Card 8.12   Intracranial Hemorrhage: Epidural ..............................133

Card 8.13   Intracranial Hemorrhage: Subdural .............................134

Card 8.14   Intracranial Hemorrhage: Subarachnoid .........................134

Card 8.15   Meningitis, Bacterial ..........................................135

Card 8.16   Meningococcemia ..............................................135

Card 8.17   Mental Status Changes: Geriatrics ..............................136

Card 8.18   Multiple Sclerosis .............................................136

Card 8.19   Myasthenia Gravis .............................................137

Card 8.20   Paralysis .....................................................137

Card 8.21   Parkinson's Disease ............................................138

Card 8.22   Peripheral Neuropathies ........................................138

Card 8.23   Seizure Disorders ..............................................139

Card 8.24   Status Epilepticus .............................................139

Card 8.25   Temporal Arteritis .............................................140

Card 8.26   Trigeminal Neuralgia ...........................................140

**Psychiatry and Behavioral Science** . . . . . . . . . . . . . . . . . . . . . . . . . . . . . . . . . . . . . . . . . .**141**

    Card 9.1  Adjustment Disorder . . . . . . . . . . . . . . . . . . . . . . . . . . . . . . . . .142

    Card 9.2  Alcohol Withdrawal . . . . . . . . . . . . . . . . . . . . . . . . . . . . . . . . . .142

    Card 9.3  Altered Mental Status: Geriatrics . . . . . . . . . . . . . . . . . . . . . . . . . . . . . .143

    Card 9.4  Bereavement, Acute . . . . . . . . . . . . . . . . . . . . . . . . . . . . . . . . . .143

    Card 9.5  Bipolar Disorder . . . . . . . . . . . . . . . . . . . . . . . . . . . . . . . . . . .144

    Card 9.6  Cocaine Abuse . . . . . . . . . . . . . . . . . . . . . . . . . . . . . . . . . . . .144

    Card 9.7  Delusional (Paranoid) Disorders . . . . . . . . . . . . . . . . . . . . . . . . . . . .145

    Card 9.8  Depression . . . . . . . . . . . . . . . . . . . . . . . . . . . . . . . . . . . . .145

    Card 9.9  Eating Disorders: Anorexia Nervosa . . . . . . . . . . . . . . . . . . . . . . . . .146

    Card 9.10  Eating Disorders: Bulimia Nervosa . . . . . . . . . . . . . . . . . . . . . . . . .146

    Card 9.11  Kübler-Ross Stages of Impending Death . . . . . . . . . . . . . . . . . . . . .147

    Card 9.12  Panic Disorder . . . . . . . . . . . . . . . . . . . . . . . . . . . . . . . . . . .147

    Card 9.13  Schizophrenia . . . . . . . . . . . . . . . . . . . . . . . . . . . . . . . . . . .148

    Card 9.14  Schizotypal Personality Disorder . . . . . . . . . . . . . . . . . . . . . . . . .148

    Card 9.15A  Suicide . . . . . . . . . . . . . . . . . . . . . . . . . . . . . . . . . . . . .149

    Card 9.15B  Suicide, Continued . . . . . . . . . . . . . . . . . . . . . . . . . . . . . . .149

**Genitourinary System** . . . . . . . . . . . . . . . . . . . . . . . . . . . . . . . . . . . . . . . . . . . . . . . . . . .**150**

    Card 10.1  Atheroembolic Renal Disease . . . . . . . . . . . . . . . . . . . . . . . . . . .151

    Card 10.2  Bladder Carcinoma . . . . . . . . . . . . . . . . . . . . . . . . . . . . . . . . .151

    Card 10.3  Diabetic Nephropathy . . . . . . . . . . . . . . . . . . . . . . . . . . . . . . .152

    Card 10.4  Epididymitis . . . . . . . . . . . . . . . . . . . . . . . . . . . . . . . . . . . .152

    Card 10.5  Glomerulonephritis . . . . . . . . . . . . . . . . . . . . . . . . . . . . . . . .153

    Card 10.6  Hematuria . . . . . . . . . . . . . . . . . . . . . . . . . . . . . . . . . . . . .153

    Card 10.7  Incontinence . . . . . . . . . . . . . . . . . . . . . . . . . . . . . . . . . . . .154

    Card 10.8  Nephrolithiasis . . . . . . . . . . . . . . . . . . . . . . . . . . . . . . . . . .154

    Card 10.9  Nephrotic Syndrome . . . . . . . . . . . . . . . . . . . . . . . . . . . . . . .155

    Card 10.10  Peyronie's Disease . . . . . . . . . . . . . . . . . . . . . . . . . . . . . . . .155

    Card 10.11  Polycystic Kidney Disease, Adult . . . . . . . . . . . . . . . . . . . . . . . . .156

    Card 10.12  Renal Cell Carcinoma . . . . . . . . . . . . . . . . . . . . . . . . . . . . . .156

    Card 10.13  Renal Failure: Acute . . . . . . . . . . . . . . . . . . . . . . . . . . . . . . .157

    Card 10.14  Renal Failure: Chronic . . . . . . . . . . . . . . . . . . . . . . . . . . . . . .157

    Card 10.15  Tubular Necrosis, Acute . . . . . . . . . . . . . . . . . . . . . . . . . . . . .158

    Card 10.16  Urinary Tract Infection . . . . . . . . . . . . . . . . . . . . . . . . . . . . . .158

**Dermatologic System** . . . . . . . . . . . . . . . . . . . . . . . . . . . . . . . . . . . . . . . . . . . . . . . . . . . .**159**

    Card 11.1  Acne Vulgaris . . . . . . . . . . . . . . . . . . . . . . . . . . . . . . . . . . .160

    Card 11.2  Collagen Vascular Disorders . . . . . . . . . . . . . . . . . . . . . . . . . . .160

    Card 11.3  Cutaneous Fungal Infections . . . . . . . . . . . . . . . . . . . . . . . . . . .161

    Card 11.4  Cutaneous Parasitic Infections . . . . . . . . . . . . . . . . . . . . . . . . . .161

    Card 11.5  Dermatitis . . . . . . . . . . . . . . . . . . . . . . . . . . . . . . . . . . . . .162

    Card 11.6  Folliculitis . . . . . . . . . . . . . . . . . . . . . . . . . . . . . . . . . . . . .162

    Card 11.7  Hidradenitis Suppurativa . . . . . . . . . . . . . . . . . . . . . . . . . . . . .163

    Card 11.8  Impetigo: Bullous . . . . . . . . . . . . . . . . . . . . . . . . . . . . . . . . .163

    Card 11.9  Impetigo: Vulgaris . . . . . . . . . . . . . . . . . . . . . . . . . . . . . . . . .164

    Card 11.10  Psoriasis . . . . . . . . . . . . . . . . . . . . . . . . . . . . . . . . . . . . .164

Card 11.11  Skin Carcinoma ....................................................165
Card 11.12  Strawberry Nevus ..................................................165
Card 11.13  Warts: Common ...................................................166
Card 11.14  Warts: Flat ........................................................166

**Hematologic System** ..........................................................**167**
Card 12.1  Anemia: Aplastic ...................................................168
Card 12.2  Anemia: Hemolytic ................................................168
Card 12.3  Anemia: Iron Deficiency ..........................................169
Card 12.4  Anemia: Megaloblastic ............................................169
Card 12.5  Anemia: Pernicious .................................................170
Card 12.6  Disseminated Intravascular Coagulation (DIC) ....................170
Card 12.7  Hemophilia .........................................................171
Card 12.8  Hodgkin's Lymphoma ..............................................171
Card 12.9  Idiopathic Thrombocytopenic Purpura (ITP) .....................172
Card 12.10  Leukemia, Acute ...................................................172
Card 12.11  Leukemia, Chronic Lymphocytic .................................173
Card 12.12  Multiple Myeloma ................................................173
Card 12.13  Non-Hodgkin's Lymphoma .......................................174
Card 12.14  Polycythemia Vera ................................................174
Card 12.15  Sickle Cell Disease ................................................175
Card 12.16  Thalassemia .......................................................175
Card 12.17  Thrombocytopenia .................................................176
Card 12.18  Von Willebrand's Disease .........................................176

**Infectious Disease** ...........................................................**177**
Card 13.1  Anthrax .............................................................178
Card 13.2  Cellulitis ...........................................................178
Card 13.3  Croup (Laryngotracheobronchitis) ...............................179
Card 13.4  Human Immunodeficiency Virus (HIV) ...........................179
Card 13.5A  Immunization Schedule: Adults .................................180
Card 13.5B  Immunization Schedule: Adults, Continued .....................180
Card 13.6  Immunization Schedule: Pediatrics ...............................181
Card 13.7  Influenza ...........................................................181
Card 13.8  Lyme Disease .......................................................182
Card 13.9  Mononucleosis, Infectious ........................................182
Card 13.10  Mumps (Epidemic Parotitis) ......................................183
Card 13.11  Neonatal Sepsis ...................................................183
Card 13.12  Osteomyelitis ......................................................184
Card 13.13  Pertussis ...........................................................184
Card 13.14  Pinworm Infection .................................................185
Card 13.15  Scarlet Fever .......................................................185
Card 13.16  Sepsis ..............................................................186
Card 13.17  Septic Arthritis ....................................................186
Card 13.18  Smallpox ...........................................................187
Card 13.19  Streptococcal Pharyngitis ........................................187

**Surgery** ..........................................................**188**

Card 14.1   Achalasia: Surgical Perspective ....................................189

Card 14.2   Appendicitis, Acute ...........................................189

Card 14.3   Atelectasis ..................................................190

Card 14.4   Burns ......................................................190

Card 14.5   Cholecystitis, Acute ..........................................191

Card 14.6   Dumping Syndrome ...........................................191

Card 14.7A  Electrolyte Disorders ..........................................192

Card 14.7B  Electrolyte Disorders, Continued .................................192

Card 14.8   Hemorrhoids .................................................193

Card 14.9   Informed Consent .............................................193

Card 14.10  Inguinal Hernia ...............................................194

Card 14.11  Pancreatic Pseudocyst .........................................194

Card 14.12  Pancreatitis, Acute ............................................195

Card 14.13  Perirectal Abscess .............................................195

Card 14.14  Peritonitis ....................................................196

Card 14.15  Preoperative Evaluation ........................................196

Card 14.16  Pseudomembranous Enterocolitis .................................197

Card 14.17  Ruptured Spleen ...............................................197

Card 14.18  Superior Vena Cava Syndrome ...................................198

Card 14.19  Testicular Torsion ..............................................198

Card 14.20  Whole Blood Transfusions .......................................199

Card 14.21  Wound Infection, Postoperative .................................199

**Pharmacology** .....................................................**200**

**SECTION A**
**Cardiovascular System Medications** .................................**201**

Card 15.1A  Antiarrhythmics ..............................................201

Card 15.1B  Antiarrhythmics, Continued .....................................201

Card 15.2   Diuretics ....................................................202

Card 15.3   Inotropes ....................................................202

Card 15.4A  Vasodilators .................................................203

Card 15.4B  Vasodilators, Continued ........................................203

Card 15.5   Autonomic Medications ........................................204

Card 15.6   Autonomic Medications: Cholinomimetics and Cholinolytics ........204

Card 15.7A  Autonomic Medications: Sympathomimetics ......................205

Card 15.7B  Autonomic Medications: Sympathomimetics, Continued ..........205

Card 15.8A  Autonomic Medications: Sympatholytics .........................206

Card 15.8B  Autonomic Medications: Sympatholytics, Continued ..............206

Card 15.8C  Autonomic Medications: Sympatholytics, Continued ..............207

Card 15.8D  Autonomic Medications: Sympatholytics, Continued ..............207

**SECTION B**
**Pulmonary System Medications** ....................................**208**

Card 15.9   Bronchodilators ..............................................208

Card 15.10A Antiasthmatics ...............................................209

Card 15.10B Antiasthmatics, Continued .....................................209

**SECTION C**
**Gastrointestinal System Medications** ...........................................210
Card 15.11A  Antacids ...........................................................210
Card 15.11B  Antacids, Continued ...............................................211
Card 15.12  Antidiarrheals .......................................................211
Card 15.13  Antiemetics .........................................................212
Card 15.14  Anticonstipation Medications .........................................212

**SECTION D**
**Musculoskeletal System Medications** ..........................................213
Card 15.15  Anti-inflammatories .................................................213
Card 15.16A  Autoimmune Diseases ..............................................214
Card 15.16B  Autoimmune Diseases, Continued ....................................214
Card 15.17  Muscle Relaxants ....................................................215

**SECTION E**
**Endocrine System Medications** ................................................216
Card 15.18A  Pituitary/Hypothalamic Hormones ...................................216
Card 15.18B  Pituitary/Hypothalamic Hormones, Continued ........................217
Card 15.19A  Adrenocorticosteroids ..............................................217
Card 15.19B  Adrenocorticosteroids, Continued ...................................218
Card 15.20  Thyroid Hormones ...................................................218
Card 15.21A  Hypoglycemic Agents ...............................................219
Card 15.21B  Hypoglycemic Agents, Continued ....................................219
Card 15.22A  Lipid Agents .......................................................220
Card 15.22B  Lipid Agents, Continued ............................................220
Card 15.23A  Osteoporosis Agents ................................................221
Card 15.23B  Osteoporosis Agents, Continued .....................................221

**SECTION F**
**Neurologic System Medications** ...............................................222
Card 15.24  Neurogenic Agents ..................................................222
Card 15.25  Antiseizure Agents ..................................................223

**SECTION G**
**Psychiatric Medications** .....................................................224
Card 15.26  Antipsychotics ......................................................224
Card 15.27  Antidepressants .....................................................225
Card 15.28  Depressants .........................................................225
Card 15.29A  Drugs of Abuse .....................................................226
Card 15.29B  Drugs of Abuse, Continued .........................................226

**SECTION H**
**Hematologic System Medications** .............................................227
Card 15.30A  Anticoagulants .....................................................227
Card 15.30B  Anticoagulants, Continued ..........................................228
Card 15.31  Thrombolytics .......................................................228
Card 15.32  Hematopoietic Agents ...............................................229

**SECTION I**
**Infectious Disease Medications** ..............................................230
Card 15.33A  Antibiotics: Bacterial Cell Wall Inhibitors ...........................230
Card 15.33B  Antibiotics: Bacterial Cell Wall Inhibitors, Continued ................231

Card 15.33C  Antibiotics: Bacterial Cell Wall Inhibitors, Continued ..............231

Card 15.34  Antibiotics: Folate Antagonists ...................................232

Card 15.35A  Antibiotics: Protein Synthesis Inhibitors .........................232

Card 15.35B  Antibiotics: Protein Synthesis Inhibitors, Continued ..............233

Card 15.35C  Antibiotics: Protein Synthesis Inhibitors, Continued ..............233

Card 15.36  Antibiotics: Nucleic Acid Inhibitors ...............................234

Card 15.37A  Antibiotics: Miscellaneous Agents ................................234

Card 15.37B  Antibiotics: Miscellaneous Agents, Continued ....................235

Card 15.38A  Antivirals ........................................................235

Card 15.38B  Antivirals, Continued ...........................................236

Card 15.38C  Antivirals, Continued ...........................................236

Card 15.39A  Antifungals ......................................................237

Card 15.39B  Antifungals, Continued ..........................................237

Card 15.40A  Antiparasitics ...................................................238

Card 15.40B  Antiparasitics, Continued .......................................238

*Appendix 1  Abbreviations* .......................................................*239*

*Appendix 2  Terminology Links* ...................................................*242*

*Index* ...........................................................................*249*

# CHAPTER 1

# Cardiovascular System

## 1.1 ANGINA PECTORIS

**Etiology:** Usually secondary to atherosclerotic heart disease, leads to a discrepancy between the myocardial requirement for oxygen and the amount delivered through the coronary arteries.

**Risk Factors:** Hyperlipidemia

**S/S:**
- Sharp, substernal CP or pressure provoked by activity and relieved by rest and/or nitrates
- +/− Elevated BP
- Gallop rhythm and apical systolic murmur (MR) during pain episode
- Pain can radiate to neck or arm
- +/− Dyspnea
- Diaphoresis
- N/V

**Dx:** Clinical dx based on characteristic complaint of CP, confirmed by stress test or angiogram

**Tx:** Nitrates for acute attack; for maintenance→activity modification, platelet inhibitor therapy (ASA), beta blockers (negative inotropic effects), calcium channel blockers (coronary artery vasodilation)

**Complications:** Can progress to MI

## 1.2 ANGINA PECTORIS, SPECIFIC TYPES

**Types:**
- Unstable
- Variant (Prinzmetal's angina)

**Etiology:**
- Unstable—accelerated or "crescendo" pattern of pain due to "complex" coronary stenosis
- Variant—secondary to large vessel spasm

**Risk Factors:** Smoking, cocaine

**S/S:**
- Unstable—any change in the pattern of previously stable symptoms, tachycardia, transient $S_3$ or $S_4$, HTN
- Variant—characterized by pain at rest and ST-segment elevation; patient is typically younger than with other types of angina

**Dx:**
- Unstable—ST-segment depression, T-wave flattening or inversion, +/− angiographic findings
- Variant—ST-segment elevation

**Tx:**
- Unstable—medical emergency, requires CCU admission, bed rest, sedation, nasal $O_2$, nitrates, anticoagulation, beta blockers; calcium channel blockers may be useful; angioplasty and/or bypass surgery may be necessary
- Variant—nitrates, either sublingual NTG or long-acting; calcium channel blockers give best long-term relief; avoid beta blockers

**Complications:**
- Unstable—acute MI, ventricular dysrhythmias, sudden death; often considered a precursor to MI, up to 30% of patients will suffer an MI within 3 months of onset
- Variant—depends on response to medications and degree of coexisting CAD

## 1.3  AORTIC ANEURYSM

**Etiology:** Atherosclerosis, HTN, infection, Marfan's syndrome, connective tissue diseases

**Risk Factors:** Smoking, male gender, advanced age, HTN

**S/S:** Depends on location—steady, gnawing pain; not affected by exertion or NTG
- Intrathoracic—cough, hoarseness, dyspnea, dysphagia, substernal or localized back pain, SUPERIOR VENA CAVA SYNDROME
- ABD—ABD/back/leg/groin/flank pain, anorexia, N/V, unilateral LE swelling, +/− ABD bruit, pulsatile ABD mass; hypotension due to leak or rupture

**Dx:**
- X-ray—abnormal mass, widened mediastinum, enlargement of aortic knob, displacement of trachea
- US—defines size and site for AAA but not useful for intrathoracic due to lungs
- CT best for intrathoracic

**Tx:** If dissection suspected, admit to CCU for emergent vascular intervention; all others, surgical referral for elective repair

**Complications:** Rupture, death, recurrence

## 1.4  ATRIOVENTRICULAR (AV) HEART BLOCKS

**Types:**
- 1st degree
- 2nd degree—Mobitz I (Wenckebach)
- 2nd degree—Mobitz II
- 3rd degree

**Etiology:**
- 1st—constant prolonged PR interval, QRS for each P wave
- Mobitz I—progressive prolongation of PR interval until QRS complex is dropped; then the AV node recovers and pattern repeats
- Mobitz II—intermittent nonconducted P wave with fixed PR intervals, usually in a constant pattern (2:1, 3:1)
- 3rd—complete dissociation between the atria and ventricles; results in haphazard contraction with each independent of the other

**S/S:**
- 1st degree—asymptomatic
- 2nd and 3rd—SOB, STOKES–ADAMS ATTACK, irregular heart rate/palpitations, JVD, hypotension, heart failure

**Dx:** ECG Shows:
- 1st—PR prolonged (> 0.2 sec) and constant, QRS for every P wave
- Mobitz I—progressive prolongation of PR until QRS dropped; R–R has progressive shortening while P–P remains constant
- Mobitz II—intermittent non-conducted P waves, PR fixed and P–P is constant
- 3rd—atrial and ventricular activity are independent, P–P constant and R–R constant while P–R has no correlation

**Tx:** Symptomatic block requires emergent treatment; definitive treatment is pacemaker

**Complications:** Heart failure, complete heart block

## 1.5  BACTERIAL ENDOCARDITIS

**Etiology:**
- Acute—*Staph. aureus*
- Subacute—*Strep. viridans*, enterococci or other Gram +/–

**Risk Factors:** Acquired valvular heart disease, congenital heart disease, prosthetic heart valves, IVDA, indwelling central venous catheters, prior endocarditis

**S/S:** Febrile illness for days to weeks, cough, dyspnea, arthralgias, arthritis, diarrhea, ABD pain or flank pain, pallor, splenomegaly, new or changed heart murmur is pathognomonic; characteristic lesions—petechiae on palate or conjunctiva, splinter hemorrhages of nails, OSLER'S NODES, JANEWAY LESIONS, ROTH'S SPOTS

**Dx:**
- CBC—acute, elevated WBC; subacute, anemia
- Blood cultures—three sets in 24 hr from different sites before starting antibiotics
- CXR, echo to confirm
- Dx based on above and Duke criteria (next card)

**Tx:** IV cephalosporin and aminoglycoside, adjust as needed once cultures and sensitivities return; 4–6 week course usually recommended

**Complications:** Valvular incompetence or obstruction, myocardial abscess, mycotic aneurysm, peripheral embolization

**Prophylaxis for At-Risk Population:**
- Dental and upper respiratory procedures—PCN PO (erythromycin in PCN allergy)
- GI or GU tract procedures—IV PCN and gentamicin (or vancomycin)

## 1.6  BACTERIAL ENDOCARDITIS: DUKE DIAGNOSTIC CRITERIA

**Criteria:** Must meet 2 major **or** 1 major and 3 minor **or** 5 minor

**Major:**
- Positive blood cultures—2 Cx drawn > 12 hr apart or all 3 Cx at least 1 hr apart
- Echo evidence of endocardial involvement

**Minor:**
- Fever >38.0°C (100.4°F)
- Preexisting CAD or IVDA
- Vascular phenomena—major arterial emboli, septic pulmonary infarcts, mycotic aneurysm, CVA, conjunctival hemorrhages, JANEWAY LESIONS
- Immunologic phenomena—OSLER'S NODES, ROTH'S SPOTS, elevated RF, glomerulonephritis
- + Blood Cx that does not meet major criteria
- + Echo findings that do not meet major criteria

## 1.7 BUERGER'S DISEASE (THROMBOANGIITIS OBLITERANS)

**Definition:** Vasculitis of small- and medium-sized arteries and veins of the extremities; more common in young men (< 45 Y/O)

**Etiology:** Unknown; definite relationship to cigarette smoking and increased incidence of HLA-B5 and HLA-A9 antigens

**S/S:**
• Reduced or absent distal pulses (wrist and ankle)
• Trophic nail changes
• Digital ulcerations
• Ischemic neuropathy
• Classic triad—intermittent claudication, Raynaud's phenomenon, and migratory superficial thrombophlebitis

**Dx:** Arteriography—smooth, tapering segmental lesions of distal vessels with surrounding collateral vessels at site of occlusion; excisional biopsy confirms diagnosis

**Tx:** Smoking cessation may improve disease with moderate success at halting disease progression; sympathectomy or amputation may be necessary for severe cases

**Complications:** Recurrences or progression of disease with repeated amputations possible; may affect cerebral, visceral, or coronary vessels

## 1.8 CARDIOGENIC SHOCK

**Note:** The most severe form of acute heart failure

**Etiology:** Post MI, hypovolemia

**S/S:** Reduced CO, hypotension, elevated pulmonary capillary wedge pressure, organ hypoperfusion, pulmonary edema, MS changes, decreased urine output, cold extremities

**Dx:**
• ECG—ST-segment elevation or depression (acute ischemic Dz) or Q waves (chronic ischemic Dz)
• Swan-Ganz cath confirms diagnosis (wedge > 18, CO < 2.2 L/kg/min)

**Tx:** Vasopressors, inotropes, diuretics, +/− PTCA or CABG (post AMI); placement of intra-aortic balloon pump may be necessary

**Complications:** Death—post AMI, approximately 70%

## 1.9A CARDIOMYOPATHY

**Types:**
- Dilated (D)—LV dilation and systolic dysfunction +/− regional wall motion abnormalities
- Restrictive (R)—normal LV size and systolic function, impaired diastolic function, +/− mild ventricular thickening
- Hypertrophic (H)—marked thickening of ventricular myocardium, small LV cavity size, hyperdynamic systolic function

**Etiology:**
- D—hyper- or hypothyroidism, tachycardia, viral infections, pregnancy, SLE, RA, toxins
- R—idiopathic, radiation, endomyocardial fibrosis, amyloidosis, carcinoid, scleroderma, post–heart transplant
- H—familial disease, autosomal dominant inheritance

**S/S:**
- D—dyspnea, orthopnea, PND, fatigue, decreased exercise tolerance, TIA, CVA, syncope
- R—SOB, fatigue, JVD, LE edema, ascites, loud $S_3$, pleural effusion, ABD fullness, nausea
- H—dyspnea, angina, syncope, CHF, sustained apical impulse, $S_4$, possible $S_3$, <u>PULSUS</u> <u>BISFERIENS</u>, coarse, crescendo-decrescendo systolic murmur over L SB, increases with inspiration, no radiation

*(continued)*

## 1.9B CARDIOMYOPATHY, Continued

**Dx:**
- ECG: D—interventricular conduction delay, LAD; R—low voltage, nonspecific ST-T wave changes, various arrhythmias; H—LVH, LAH, LAD
- CXR: D—cardiomegaly, pulmonary edema, pleural effusion; R—unremarkable, possible small cardiac shadow; H—+/− cardiomegaly
- Echo: D—all four chambers dilated; decreased LV systolic function; R—abnormal diastolic function, normal ventricular size and systolic function; H—marked LVH, systolic anterior motion of mitral apparatus, MR, dynamic gradient

**Tx:**
- D—control excess body water (diuretics), decrease afterload (vasodilators, ACE inhibitors), augment contractility (digoxin)
- R—treat underlying disorders, standard CHF treatment, avoid dehydration; heart transplant may be necessary as a last resort
- H—lifestyle modification, meds (beta blockers, calcium channel blockers, disopyramide), pacemaker

**Complications:** CHF, sudden cardiac death

## 1.10 CONGENITAL HEART DEFECTS: ATRIAL SEPTAL DEFECT

**Etiology:** 3 types:
- Ostium secundum defect—in midportion of the atrial septum
- Ostium primum defect—located in the low atrial septum
- Sinus venosus defect—at the junction of the R atrium and superior or inferior vena cava

**S/S:**
- Asymptomatic if small or moderate
- Large defects—exertional dyspnea, palpitations, cardiac failure, prominent R ventricular heave, cyanosis (infants)
- Murmur—loud systolic ejection murmur in 2–3 ICS, middiastolic rumble at the lower R sternal border, wide split $S_2$

**Dx:**
- ECG—RAD, RVH, +/− R BBB
- CXR—large pulmonary artery, increased pulmonary vascularity and enlarged R atrium and/or ventricle, small aortic knob
- Echo is diagnostic—identifies exact location of the defect

**Tx:** Surgical correction

**Complications:** Pulmonary HTN, cardiac arrhythmia, heart failure

## 1.11 CONGENITAL HEART DEFECTS: COARCTATION OF THE AORTA

**Etiology:** Congenital localized narrowing of the aortic arch just distal to the origin of the L subclavian artery

**S/S:**
- Higher BP in the upper than lower extremities
- Absent or weak femoral pulses
- Strong arterial pulsations in the neck and suprasternal notch
- Murmur—harsh, late systolic ejection murmur best heard at the base and posteriorly

**Dx:**
- ECG—LVH
- CXR—rib notching (scalloping), dilated L subclavian artery, poststenotic aortic dilation, +/− LVH (RVH in the neonate)
- Cardiac cath or aortography are diagnostic

**Tx:** Balloon angioplasty with or without stent placement; surgical resection may be necessary; antibiotic prophylaxis is recommended

**Complications:** Cardiac failure, HTN, ruptured aorta, infective endocarditis, CVA

## 1.12 CONGENITAL HEART DEFECTS: PATENT DUCTUS ARTERIOSUS

**Etiology:** Embryonic ductus arteriosus fails to close normally, persists as a shunt between the L pulmonary artery and the aorta

**S/S:**
- May be asymptomatic if small
- Large defect—CHF, slow growth, repeated lower respiratory tract infections, SOB, dyspnea on exertion, cyanosis
- Bounding pulses are common, wide pulse pressure and decreased diastolic BP
- Murmur—"machinery-like murmur"; a continuous, rough murmur at 2nd L ICS, accentuated in late systole (at $S_2$), trails off during diastole

**Dx:**
- ECG—L or biventricular hypertrophy
- CXR—+/− LVH/LAH, prominent pulmonary artery, aorta, and L atrium
- Echo, cardiac cath, angiography to diagnose

**Tx:** Indomethacin is often effective in the neonate, surgical correction needed in persistent cases

**Complications:** Cardiac failure, CHF, pulmonary HTN

## 1.13 CONGENITAL HEART DEFECTS: PULMONARY STENOSIS

**Etiology:** Congenital obstructive disorder that limits pulmonary blood flow

**S/S:**
- May be asymptomatic in mild cases
- Moderate to severe cases—exertional dyspnea, syncope, CP, RV failure, palpable parasternal heave, +/− R-sided $S_4$
- Murmur—harsh, loud, systolic ejection murmur with prominent thrill at L2–3 ICS
- In severe cases, may present as emergency in immediate neonatal period

**Dx:**
- ECG—RAD, RVH, peaked P waves
- CXR—+/− prominent R atrial or ventricular shadow, gross cardiomegaly in severe cases, possible poststenotic dilation of pulmonary artery with normal or decreased vascular markings

**Tx:** Percutaneous balloon valvuloplasty, surgical repair or replacement

**Complications:** Sudden death, HF in 20–30 Y/O group

## 1.14 CONGENITAL HEART DEFECTS: TETRALOGY OF FALLOT

**Etiology:** 4 defects:
- VSD with anterior malalignment
- R ventricular outflow obstruction (PS)
- RVH
- "Overriding" large ascending aorta

**S/S:**
- Retarded growth and development, cyanosis, clubbing, dyspnea with exertion that improves with squatting, prominent RV heave, +/– precordial thrill, "TET SPELLS"
- Murmur—loud systolic ejection murmur at L upper SB

**Dx:**
- ECG—RVH, R atrial dilation, RAD
- CXR—small heart size or "boot"-shaped cardiac shadow due to R-sided enlargement, decreased pulmonary vascular markings
- CBC—polycythemia

**Tx:** "Tet spells"—supplemental oxygen, vagal maneuvers, MSO4, vasoconstrictors, beta blockers, volume, "knee-chest" position; surgical repair is definitive treatment

**Complications:** HF, sudden death

## 1.15 CONGENITAL HEART DEFECTS: VENTRICULAR SEPTAL DEFECT

**Etiology:** Persistent opening or openings in the intraventricular septum, resulting in failure of fusion with the aortic septum

**S/S:**
- SOB, dyspnea, CP, cyanosis with large defects, +/– RV heave
- Small—early systolic murmur or diamond-shaped murmur; systolic thrill +/– pulmonary HTN, AR
- Large—loud, harsh holosystolic murmur in the L3–4 ICS along sternum, +/– middiastolic flow murmur and $S_3$ at apex

**Dx:**
- ECG—NSR +/– RVH/LVH
- CXR—L atrial and pulmonary artery enlargement, increased pulmonary vascularity
- Echo or cardiac cath is diagnostic

**Tx:** Surgical correction; antibiotic prophylaxis throughout life

**Complications:** CHF, infective endocarditis

## 1.16A CONGESTIVE HEART FAILURE

**Etiology:** Classified as systolic or diastolic, precipitating causes vary
- Systolic—ischemic heart disease (CAD, MI); idiopathic, congenital, or acquired valvular disorders; HTN; amyloidosis; hemochromatosis; sarcoidosis; inflammatory myocarditis; metabolic abnormalities; toxins
- Diastolic—systemic HTN, cardiomyopathies

**S/S:** Classified as right- or left-sided:
- R sided—LE edema worse with standing and improved with elevation of legs, ABD discomfort, nausea, increased jugular venous pressure, hepatomegaly, +/– ascites and CP
- L sided—dyspnea, orthopnea, PND, fatigue, lethargy, +/– CP, rales, dullness to percussion at bases, L $S_3$ (systolic dysfunction), L $S_4$ (diastolic dysfunction), LV heave

**Dx:**
- ECG—nonspecific changes, arrhythmias, LVH
- CXR—cardiomegaly, pulmonary vascular congestion, +/– pleural effusion
- Echo—evaluates cardiac output and ejection fraction, determines type of failure (systolic/diastolic)
- Labs—CBC, RFT, LFT, TFT, PFT, UA, electrolytes
- Swan-Ganz cath—confirms diagnosis

*(continued)*

## 1.16B CONGESTIVE HEART FAILURE, Continued

**Tx:**
- General—determine cause, search for correctable conditions, and eliminate contributing factors (limit salt intake, exercise regularly, stop smoking, lipid control, weight loss, avoid ETOH, drugs)
- Acute care—reduce cardiac workload (bed rest and sedation); control excessive fluid retention (decrease sodium intake and diuretics); reduce afterload (with vasodilators, ACE inhibitors, NTG); enhance myocardial contractility (digoxin, sympathomimetics)

**Complications:** Unless there is a reversible cause, HF is a progressive disorder with high morbidity and mortality

## 1.17 CORONARY ARTERY DISEASE

**Definition:** Progressive degenerative process; begins in childhood and manifests in middle to late adulthood as acute coronary syndrome (unstable angina, AMI), or chronic ischemic heart disease (chronic stable angina, ischemic cardiomyopathy)

**Etiology:** Atherosclerotic plaque formation, infection, rheumatic vasculitis, congenital anomalies, coronary artery aneurysm, infections (rare)

**Risk Factors:** HTN, hyperlipidemia, diabetes, smoking, age, male gender, family history, obesity, physical inactivity

**S/S:** Depend on severity—exertional CP and pressure, LEVINE'S SIGN, exertional SOB, fatigue, near syncope, nausea, diaphoresis

**Dx:**
- ECG—ST-segment depression = myocardial ischemia; ST-segment elevation = acute myocardial injury; Q wave = prior MI
- Stress test—to demonstrate significant CAD
- Angio—"gold standard," assesses patency of vessel

**Tx:** Lifestyle modification (diet, exercise, stop smoking, lipid-lowering medications); NTG PRN; aggressive control of HTN and DM; medications (ASA, beta blockers, ACE inhibitors, statins); PTCA (angioplasty +/− stenting) or CABG

**Complications:** MI, sudden cardiac death, CHF, valvular heart disease, dysrhythmias

## 1.18 DEEP VENOUS THROMBOSIS

**Etiology:** Thrombus formation in the deep veins of the leg or pelvis; VIRCHOW'S TRIAD indicates those at higher risk

**S/S:** Unilateral limb swelling, pain and/or tightness, edema, increased vascular markings distal to the DVT, +/− fever, HOMANS' SIGN

**Dx:** Clinical diagnosis—confirmed by elevated D-dimer and duplex Doppler US

**Tx:**
- Prophylaxis in at-risk populations (ambulation, compressive stockings, compression devices)
- Anticoagulation (SQ heparin or low-molecular-weight heparin, PO warfarin, ASA): 1st DVT = full anticoagulation (INR 2–3) for 4–6 months; 2nd DVT = full anticoagulation for 12 months; 3rd DVT = anticoagulation for life
- Consider vena cava filter if patient is not a candidate for anticoagulation
- Symptomatic treatment for DVT = analgesia, compression, heat

**Complications:** PE, CVA, TROUSSEAU'S SIGN

# 1.19 DYSRHYTHMIAS: BRADYDYSRHYTHMIAS

**Etiology:**
- Functional—abnormalities resulting from autonomic or pharmacological causes
- Structural—conduction system disease (fibrosis of SA or AV node, amyloidosis, sarcoidosis, ischemia or infarction, congenital complete heart block)

**S/S:** HR < 60 bpm, dizziness/light-headedness, confusion, fatigue, syncope/near-syncope, angina, CHF

**Dx:**
- ECG—evaluate presence and pattern of P waves and their relation to QRS complexes
- Holter monitoring—may be necessary for intermittent disturbances

**Tx:**
- Asymptomatic—no treatment required
- Symptomatic—discontinue any medications that slow conduction, treat ischemia/infarction, atropine, implantable pacemaker

**Complications:** Progression of heart block, cardiogenic shock, death

# 1.20 DYSRHYTHMIAS: BRADYDYSRHYTHMIAS, SPECIFIC TYPES

**Types:**
- Sinus bradycardia (SB)
- Sinus nodal dysfunction (SND)
- Heart block (1, 2-I, 2-II, 3)

**Etiology:**
- SB—increased vagal tone, medications, hypothyroidism, hypothermia, advanced liver disease, intrinsic SA nodal disease
- SND—amyloidosis, fibrosis of SA node, SICK SINUS SYNDROME
- 1—idiopathic
- 2-I—vagal tone
- 2-II—structural disease
- 3—MI

**Dx:** ECG shows:
- SB—normal P wave, P wave for every QRS, rate < 60 bpm
- SND—bradycardia, intermittent prolonged sinus pauses, complete sinus arrest, +/− junctional or ventricular escape rhythms

- 1—fixed prolongation of PR interval (>200 msec)
- 2-I—PR progressively prolongs until a P wave fails to conduct (QRS dropped)
- 2-II—PR interval consistent for all conducted beats, occasionally 1 or more QRS dropped
- 3—complete dissociation between P wave and QRS. QRS wide; usually nodal or ventricular escape rhythm

**Tx:**
- SB—treat underlying cause, atropine, pacemaker if symptomatic and refractory to other treatments
- SND and 2-I—usually requires no treatment
- SND 2-II and 3—require implantable pacemaker

## 1.21 DYSRHYTHMIAS: TACHYDYSRHYTHMIAS

**Etiology:** Prior MI, LV aneurysm, cardiomyopathy, valvular disease, hypertrophic heart disease, ↑ catecholamines (pain, fear, anxiety), hyper- or hypokalemia, hypomagnesemia, hypocalcemia, hyperthyroidism, drugs, medications

**S/S:** Palpitations, light-headedness/dizziness, syncope, CP, dyspnea, +/− hypotension, rales

**Dx:** ECG:
- Narrow QRS (< 0.120 sec)—almost always SVT
- Wide QRS (> 0.120 sec)—either VT or SVT with aberrant conduction
- Assess regularity and presence/absence of P waves to diagnose specific dysrhythmia

**Tx:**
- Goal—control ventricular rate and terminate and prevent recurrence of dysrhythmia
- Vagal maneuvers
- AV-nodal blocking drugs
- Antiarrhythmic medications
- Cardioversion/defibrillation
- Radiofrequency ablation often curative

**Complications:** Sudden cardiac death, cardiogenic shock, recurrence

Takotsubo cardiomyopathy
Non-ischemic cardiomyopathy

## 1.22A  DYSRHYTHMIAS: TACHYDYSRHYTHMIAS, SPECIFIC TYPES

**Types:**
- Sinus tach (ST)
- Ectopic atrial tach (EAT)
- Multifocal atrial tach (MAT)
- Atrial fibrillation (AFb)
- Atrial flutter (AFl)
- AV node reentry tach (AVN)
- AV reentry tach (AV)
- Ventricular tach (VT)

**Etiology:**
- ST—response to some physiological stimulus
- EAT—may occur in absence of identifiable precipitant
- MAT—severe lung disease
- AFb—rheumatic heart disease, HTN, CHF, advanced age
- AFl—macro reentrant circuit in the atrium
- AVN—results from small reentrant loop within the AV node, usually initiated by a PAC
- AV—large reentrant loop with 1 limb including AV node and the other an accessory pathway (WPW), usually initiated by a premature beat
- VT—produced by reentrant circuit located in either ventricle, usually due to acute myocardial ischemia, MI, cardiomyopathy, hypokalemia, hypomagnesemia, drug toxicity, or congenital abnormality

*(continued)*

## 1.22B  DYSRHYTHMIAS: TACHYDYSRHYTHMIAS, SPECIFIC TYPES, Continued

**Dx:** ECG:
- ST—normal P waves, rate rarely > 200 bpm
- EAT—P waves inverted in inferior leads, upright in aVR
- MAT—irregularly irregular rhythm with > 3 different P-wave morphologies and > 3 PR intervals
- AFb—no P waves, irregularly irregular rhythm, ventricular rate 100–170 bpm
- AFl—flutter waves, atrial rate 250–350/ventricular rate 100–170 bpm
- AVN—rate 170–200 bpm, regular rhythm, retrograde or absent P wave
- AV—(WPW) delta waves in NSR, may be narrow or wide QRS
- VT—regular, wide QRS, +/– P waves but no association with QRS, +/– TORSADE DE POINTES

**Tx:**
- ST—treat only if symptomatic, correct underlying cause, AV nodal blocking medications PRN
- EAT—beta or calcium channel blockers
- MAT—verapamil, treat underlying lung disease
- AFb—rate control, stroke prevention, restoration and maintenance of sinus rhythm
- AFl—treat as AFb; radiofrequency ablation may be curative
- AVN/AV—AV-nodal blocking agents, radiofrequency ablation is curative
- VT—countershock, Rx

**Complications:** Progression to ventricular tachydysrhythmias, heart failure, death

## 1.23A  ECG ESSENTIALS

**Rate:** Large boxes—300, 150, 100, 75, 60, 50; count between QRS complexes

**Axis:**
- Normal—QRS positive in both I and aVF
- Extreme R deviation—QRS negative in I and aVF
- L deviation—QRS negative in aVF and positive in I
- R deviation—QRS negative in I
- L vector—QRS positive in I
- Downward vector—QRS positive in aVF

**Hypertrophy:**
- R atrial—large (> 0.12 msec) biphasic P wave with tall initial component
- RV—R > S in $V_1$, R progressively smaller in $V_1$ through $V_6$, S persists in $V_3$ and $V_6$, wide QRS
- L atrial—large (> 0.12 msec) biphasic P wave with tall terminal component
- LV—S in $V_1$ plus R in $V_3 \geq 35$ mm, LAD, wide QRS, inverted T waves

**Location:** Leads that identify which anatomical portion of the LV is injured
- Anterior—Q wave in $V_1$ through $V_5$
- Lateral—Q wave in I, aVL, $V_6$
- Posterior—large R wave in $V_1$, significant Q wave in $V_6$
- Inferior—Q wave in II, III, and aVF

*(continued)*

## 1.23B  ECG ESSENTIALS, Continued

**Non-Q-Wave Infarction:** Subendocardial ischemia
- Early ECG—depressed ST segment and inverted T waves
- Late ECG—ST returns to baseline and inverted T waves

**Q-Wave Infarction:** Transmural ischemia
- Early ECG—ST-segment elevation, upright T waves
- Late ECG—large Q wave, ST segment remains elevated, inverted T waves

**Electrolyte Effects:**
- Hyperkalemia—wide, flat P wave; wide QRS, peaked T waves
- Hypokalemia—flat T wave, U wave
- Hypercalcemia—short Q-T
- Hypocalcemia—long QT

## 1.24 HEART SOUNDS

**Loud $S_1$:** Mitral stenosis

**Variable $S_1$:** Atrial fibrillation, atrioventricular dissociation

**Loud $A_2$:** HTN

**Soft $A_2$:** Aortic stenosis

**Loud $P_2$:** Pulmonary HTN

**Fixed, Split $S_2$:** ASD

**Paradoxical Split $S_2$:** LBBB, severe aortic stenosis, PDA

**Widely Split $S_2$ with Normal Variation:** RBBB

**$S_3$:** LV dysfunction

**$S_4$:** HTN, aortic stenosis, hypertrophic cardiomyopathy

**Early Systolic Ejection Click:** Bicuspid aortic valve, pulmonary stenosis, pulmonary HTN

**Midsystolic Click:** Mitral valve prolapse

**Opening Snap:** Mitral stenosis

**Pericardial Knock:** Constrictive pericarditis

**Pericardial Friction Rub:** Pericarditis

## 1.25 HYPERTENSION

**Etiology:**
- Primary (essential)—idiopathic
- Secondary—has an identifiable cause (OCP use, renal disease, primary hyperaldosteronism, pheochromocytoma, coarctation of the aorta, pregnancy-induced, hyperthyroidism, drug use, Cushing's disease, hyperparathyroidism, carcinoid syndrome, hypothyroidism)

**S/S:**
- Primary—may be asymptomatic early in disease
- Secondary—depends on underlying cause
- Late findings—retinal changes per KEITH–WAGNER–BARKER CLASSIFICATION, LVH, CHF, PVD, signs of end-organ damage if in crisis

**Dx:** Based on 3 consecutive readings above 140/90; any of the following: PRN CBC, BUN/creatinine, chemistries UA, lipid panel, ECG, ABD CT/MRI, IVP, renal US, echocardiogram

**Tx:** "Stepped-care" approach:
- Non-Rx if diastolic less than 95—treat with weight loss, salt/cholesterol restriction, exercise
- Rx—start with primary class, add secondary as needed
- Young pt—sympatholytic (primary); ACE inhibitor (secondary)
- Middle-aged pt—alpha blocker, ACE inhibitor, calcium channel blocker
- + angina—calcium channel blocker
- + CHF—ACE inhibitor
- Elderly pt—ACE inhibitor (CHF), calcium channel blocker (CAD), alpha blocker (secondary)
- Obese pt—start with diuretic, then add primary according to age PRN

**Complications:** Atherosclerosis, LV hypertrophy, LV diastolic dysfunction, CHF, aortic aneurysm, aortic dissection, CVA/TIA, nephrosclerosis, renal insufficiency; untreated or undertreated HTN shortens life span by 10–20 years

## 1.26 HYPERTENSION, SPECIFIC TYPES

**Types:**
- Portal (P)
- Pulmonary (PUL)
- Malignant (M)

**Etiology:**
- P—increased resistance to blood flow through portal vein
- PUL—primary (idiopathic) or secondary (PE, CHF, interstitial disease)
- M—fibrinoid necrosis of arterioles of the kidney

**S/S:**
- P—ascites, splenomegaly, hepatic encephalopathy, portosystemic shunting, jaundice, edema, gynecomastia, palmar erythema, spider angiomas
- PUL—dyspnea, fatigue, CP, syncope, hemoptysis, hoarseness, RAYNAUD'S PHENOMENON, COR PULMONALE
- M—persistent diastolic BP > 120, papilledema, evidence of renal involvement

**Dx:**
- P—clinical Dx, may measure portal vein pressure to confirm
- PUL—CXR ($\uparrow$ hilum), ECG (RAD, RVH, RV strain), echo (best test to estimate PA pressure)
- M—renal insufficiency (proteinuria, microscopic hematuria, granular casts)

**Tx:**
- P—treat underlying cause and manage acute problems PRN
- PUL—treat underlying disorder, lung transplant if other Tx fails
- M—aggressive lowering of BP and management of renal failure

**Complications:**
- P—esophageal varices may lead to massive hematemesis, hepatorenal syndrome, hepatopulmonary syndrome, bacterial peritonitis (secondary to infection of ascitic fluid)
- PUL—mean survival is 3 years from Dx due to advanced stage at time of presentation; end stage results in death due to RV failure or arrhythmia
- M—mortality 50% within 6 months and nearly 100% by 1 year if untreated; may result in complete renal failure necessitating dialysis, possibly for remainder of life

## 1.27A MURMURS

|  | AS | AR | MS | MR | MVP | PS | TR | COA | ASD | VSD | PDA |
|---|---|---|---|---|---|---|---|---|---|---|---|
| **Heart Sounds** | Paradoxic split $S_2$, $S_4$ | Normal, poss loud A2 | Accent $S_1$ | Low-pitched $S_3$ |  | Delayed, soft $S_2$ |  |  |  | Loud $S_2$ | Loud $S_2$ |
| **Frequency** | Harsh, rough | High-pitched blowing | Low-pitched rumbling | High-pitched blowing; musical |  | High pitched |  | Harsh | Rumble |  |  |
| **Timing** | Late systolic | Diastolic | Beginning of diastole | Midsystolic | Midsystolic | Late systolic | Holosystolic | Systolic | Midsystolic | Pansystolic |  |
| **Type** | Eject click | Decrescendo | Loud opening snap | Loud click | Midsystolic click | Ejection |  |  | Ejection |  | Loud, cont |
| **Location** | R 2 ICS | L SB 3–4 ICS | Apex L SB | Apex | Apex | L 2 ICS | L lower SB | Back | Pulm area | Apex L SB | Pulm area |
| **Other** | Use bell, pt leans forward | Diaphragm wide pulse press dia BP < 60 | Bell L lat recumbent position | Diaphragm |  |  | Pulsatile liver |  |  |  |  |

*(continued)*

## 1.27B MURMURS, Continued

|  | AS | AR | MS | MR | MVP | PS | TR | COA | ASD | VSD | PDA |
|---|---|---|---|---|---|---|---|---|---|---|---|
| **Radiation** | Neck vessels |  |  | L axilla | Varies |  |  |  |  |  |  |
| **Thrill** | Midsystolic aortic area sternal notch |  | Mid-diastolic or pre-systolic | Systolic over PMI |  |  |  |  | L 4 ICS |  |  |
| **Lift** | LV | LV apical impulse to axilla |  | RV |  |  |  |  |  |  |  |
| **Palpation** | Heave PMI to L lower MCL | Apical forceful, displaced to L and lower | Tapping over PMI RV pulse L 3–5 ICS | Brisk PMI |  |  |  |  | Pulm artery pulsation |  |  |
| **Inspection** | Sustained PMI; prom atrial fill wave | Increased PMI L MCL and lower | Precordial bulge | Prominent hyper-dynamic apical impulse to L MCL |  |  |  |  |  |  |  |

## 1.28 MYOCARDIAL INFARCTION

**Etiology:** Occlusive thrombosis, coronary vasospasm

**S/S:** Substernal crushing CP, SOB, nausea, diaphoresis, near-syncope, hypotension, arrhythmias, pulmonary edema

**Dx:**
- ECG—normal does not rule out MI; ST-segment elevation = ST-segment elevation MI; ST-segment depression and/or T-wave inversion = unstable angina or non-ST-segment elevation MI; Q wave = prior MI
- Cardiac enzymes—presence of CK-MB, troponin I or troponin T = MI; absence of enzymes = unstable angina

**Tx:**
- Initial—ASA, NTG, beta blockers, oxygen, MSO4, consider thrombolysis in ST-segment elevation MI if presents < 12 hr from onset
- Long term—medications to treat specific conditions, angioplasty or CABG

**Complications:**
- Immediate—arrhythmias, HF, cardiogenic shock, sudden death, CHF
- Delayed—muscle rupture, pericarditis, DRESSLER'S SYNDROME, emboli
- Remote—ventricular aneurysm

## 1.29 MYOCARDITIS

**Etiology:** Idiopathic (viral), acute rheumatic fever, toxins, drugs (hypersensitivity), Lyme disease, systemic diseases (collagen vascular, autoimmune, or granulomatous diseases)

**S/S:**
- New onset CHF in healthy young person, commonly with flu-like symptoms 2–3 weeks before onset (idiopathic)
- Palpitations, syncope, tachycardia, dyspnea, pericardial friction rub, sudden cardiac death, dysrhythmias, pleural-pericardial CP, gallop rhythm

**Dx:**
- ECG—sinus tach, non-specific ST–T changes, AV blocks, dysrhythmias
- Labs—↑ CPK and troponin (only in acute phase); ↑ ESR

**Tx:** Supportive—restriction of strenuous physical activity, standard CHF treatment if needed, +/− steroids; antibiotics if a specific pathogen can be isolated; avoid NSAIDs

**Complications:** CHF, sudden death, giant cell myocarditis, dilated cardiomyopathy

## 1.30 PERICARDIAL DISORDERS

**Types:**
- Pericardial effusion (E)
- Pericardial tamponade (T)

**Etiology:** May occur due to any disease that causes pericarditis—trauma, acute pericarditis, wall rupture, aortic dissection, cardiac surgery, hypothyroidism, neoplasm, uremia

**S/S:**
- Tachycardia, hypotension, dyspnea/SOB, JVD, distant cardiac sounds, LE edema, hepatomegaly, ascites
- T—increased area of cardiac dullness, orthopnea, +/− pericardial friction rub, palpitations, CP, ALOC, agitation, KUSSMAUL'S SIGN, EWART'S SIGN, PULSUS PARADOXUS, BECK'S TRIAD

**Dx:**
- Echocardiogram—2 echo signals behind the LV in the region of the posterior cardiac wall, impaired ventricular diastolic filling
- CXR—cardiomegaly, globular cardiac contour ("water bottle" appearance due to effusion)
- ECG—low-voltage QRS; T = ELECTRICAL ALTERNANS

**Tx:** Pericardiocentesis, IV fluid, support, recurrent cases may require pericardial window

**Complications:**
- E—pericardial tamponade, infection
- T—sudden death, infection

## 1.31 PERICARDITIS

**Etiology:** Usually secondary to an infection, MI, trauma, neoplasms; other causes include autoimmune diseases, radiation, medications, renal diseases, amyloidosis, sarcoidosis

**S/S:** Pleuritic and postural CP, substernal, +/− radiation to neck, shoulders, back or epigastrium; dyspnea, fevers, myalgias, fatigue, pericardial friction rub (scratching, high-pitched, superficial sound)

**Dx:**
- ECG—ST-T changes, PR depression; characteristic progression = general ST-segment elevation → return to baseline → T-wave inversion
- CXR—cardiomegaly, +/− pulmonary vascular changes
- Echo—shows effusion

**Tx:** Antibiotics only if pathogen can be isolated, otherwise symptomatic treatment; pain responds well to high-dose ASA

**Complications:** Cardiac tamponade, pericardial effusion

## 1.32 PERIPHERAL VASCULAR DISEASE

**Etiology:** Atherosclerotic obstructive disease

**Risk Factors:** Hyperlipidemia, diabetes, smoking, hypertension, advanced age, male gender

**S/S:** INTERMITTENT CLAUDICATION, decreased or absent peripheral pulses, arterial bruits, ulcerations, pallor of feet with elevation or exertion, muscle atrophy, hair loss, thickened toenails, skin fissures, shiny skin, gangrene, LERICHE'S SYNDROME

**Dx:** Clinical diagnosis based on Fontaine classification (Card 1.33); noninvasive tests—ANKLE BRACHIAL INDEX (ABI), US, MRI; angiogram should be done only if surgery is planned

**Tx:** Correct risk factors, regular exercise (will increase collateral circulation), meticulous foot care to prevent wounds, antiplatelet or vasoactive medications, surgical revascularization for severe cases, amputation

**Complications:** Acute arterial occlusion, arterial aneurysm, gangrene, amputation

## 1.33  PERIPHERAL VASCULAR DISEASE: FONTAINE DIAGNOSTIC CLASSIFICATION

**Stage I:** Asymptomatic

**Stage II:** Intermittent Claudication

**Stage III:** Resting and Nocturnal Pain

**Stage IV:** Necrosis, Gangrene

## 1.34  RHEUMATIC HEART DISEASE

**Etiology:** Sequela to hemolytic streptococcal infection

**S/S:** Fever, dyspnea, tachycardia, MR, AR, pericarditis, arthritis, painless nodules, ERYTHEMA MARGINATUM, SYDENHAM'S CHOREA

**Dx:**
- Elevated ESR, Duckett-Jones criteria (Card 1.35) on P/E (2 major or 1 major and 2 minor criteria)
- Echo—valvular dysfunction and evidence of myocardial and/or pericardial involvement

**Tx:** Antibiotics to treat initial infection; treat HF symptomatically; NSAIDs or ASA PRN joint pain; antibiotic prophylaxis for life

**Complications:** CHF, pericarditis, acquired valvular heart disease, rheumatic pneumonitis

## 1.35  RHEUMATIC HEART DISEASE: DUCKETT-JONES DIAGNOSTIC CRITERIA

**Criteria:** Require 2 major or 1 major and 2 minor findings:

**Major**
- Carditis
- Polyarthritis
- Sydenham's chorea
- Erythema marginatum
- Subcutaneous nodules

**Minor**
- Previous rheumatic fever
- Arthralgias
- Fever
- Elevated ESR/CRP/WBC
- Prolonged PR interval

## 1.36  SUDDEN CARDIAC DEATH

**Etiology:** CAD, prior MI, valvular heart disease, hypertrophic heart disease, dilated cardiomyopathy, infiltrative heart disease, prolonged QT syndrome, congenital heart disease, preexcitation syndrome, cardiac tumors

**S/S:** Cardiac arrest

**Dx:**
- ECG—old or evolving MI, preexcitation, long QT
- Labs—electrolytes, CPK, troponin

**Tx:**
- Acute—CPR, full ACLS treatment
- If patient resuscitated—treat any reversible causes, cardiac angioplasty or CABG, implantable cardioverter/defibrillator

**Complications:** Death, recurrent SCD, neurological injury, infectious complications due to prolonged intubations

## 1.37 VALVULAR DISEASES: AORTIC REGURGITATION

**Etiology:** Rheumatic fever, congenital bicuspid valve, infective endocarditis, HTN, aortitis, trauma, SLE, RA, Marfan's syndrome, seronegative spondyloarthropathies

**S/S:**
- Angina, syncope, SOB, orthopnea, paroxysmal nocturnal dyspnea, wide pulse pressure, QUINCKE'S PULSE, DUROZIEZ'S MURMUR, CORRIGAN'S PULSE, DE MUSSET'S SIGN, TRAUBE'S SIGN, MULLER'S SIGN, HILL'S SIGN
- Murmur—high pitched, diastolic decrescendo

**Dx:**
- ECG—LVH
- CXR—cardiomegaly with prominent LV
- Echo—evaluates aortic root dilation and early closure of mitral valve

**Tx:** Vasodilators may postpone surgery in asymptomatic patient; surgical repair/replacement is curative; transplant if LV function severely impaired; antibiotic prophylaxis for life recommended

**Complications:** CHF

## 1.38 VALVULAR DISEASES: AORTIC STENOSIS

**Etiology:** Congenital valvular disease (bicuspid valve), acquired disease (rheumatic heart disease, senile degeneration), secondary to other processes (peripheral pulmonary stenosis, hypercalcemia)

**S/S:**
- Classic triad—dyspnea, chest pain, syncope
- +/− palpable $S_4$, systolic thrill over upper SB
- Murmur—low-pitched, harsh, crescendo-decrescendo, systolic murmur, loudest at 2nd L ICS, +/− radiation to carotids

**Dx:**
- ECG—LVH
- CXR—cardiomegaly, calcification of aortic valve, dilation of aorta distal to stenotic lesion
- Echo is diagnostic—level and severity of obstruction, +/− diastolic dysfunction

**Tx:** Surgical replacement is "gold standard," anticoagulation, +/− balloon valvuloplasty; antibiotic prophylaxis recommended for all patients

**Complications:** Sudden death (up to 20% of all cases), arrhythmias

## 1.39 VALVULAR DISEASES: MITRAL REGURGITATION

**Etiology:** Rheumatic heart disease, myxomatous degeneration of mitral valve, papillary muscle dysfunction, ruptured chordae tendineae; mitral valve prolapse most common for isolated MR

**S/S:**
- Palpitations, dyspnea, fatigue, orthopnea, atrial fibrillation, pulmonary edema, RV heave, brisk carotid upstroke with prominent $S_3$, apical systolic thrill
- Murmur—pansystolic, maximal at apex, radiating to axilla/base; possible crescendo to $S_2$, +/− midsystolic click

**Dx:**
- ECG—atrial fib, L atrial enlargement, bifid P wave in lead II, +/− LVH
- CXR—enlarged L atrium (straightening of L heart border), LVH, +/− CHF
- Echo—L atrial enlargement and Doppler measurement of regurgitation jet; also evaluates valvular apparatus

**Tx:** Afterload reduction (ACE inhibitor or nitrates plus hydralazine), diuretics, digoxin; prosthetic valve replacement in young or tissue valve in elderly is curative; prophylaxis against endocarditis is recommended for all

**Complications:** R-sided heart failure, endocarditis, systemic emboli

## 1.40 VALVULAR DISEASES: MITRAL STENOSIS

**Etiology:** Rheumatic heart disease is predominant cause; also may be congenital, iatrogenic, or due to RA, SLE, or carcinoid heart disease

**S/S:**
- Exertional dyspnea, PND, orthopnea, hemoptysis, embolic events, CP, fatigue, ascites, edema, R parasternal heave
- Classic triad—localized middiastolic low-pitched rumbling murmur with opening snap and loud $S_1$

**Dx:**
- ECG—notched P waves, RVH, L atrial enlargement, atrial fibrillation
- CXR—straightening of L cardiac border, dilated pulmonary arteries, pulmonary vascular congestion
- Echo—classic "hockey-stick" and calcified appearance of anterior mitral valve leaflet, narrowing of mitral valve orifice and L atrial enlargement

**Tx:** Beta or calcium channel blockers to slow heart rate, diuretics, anticoagulation or ASA, open mitral commissurotomy, valve replacement, balloon valvuloplasty, antibiotic prophylaxis for life is essential

**Complications:** Secondary to prosthetic valves—thrombosis, paravalvular leak, endocarditis, degenerative changes

## 1.41  VALVULAR DISEASES: MITRAL VALVE PROLAPSE

**Etiology:** Myxomatous transformation of mitral valve, Marfan's syndrome; typical patient is thin female 14–30 Y/O

**S/S:**
- Nonspecific chest pain, dyspnea, fatigue, palpitations, S/S of MR
- Murmur—mid- to late-systolic click, high-pitched late-systolic crescendo-decrescendo at apex; accentuated with standing

**Dx:**
- ECG—biphasic or inverted T waves in II, III, aVF
- Echo is diagnostic

**Tx:** Vasodilators, intra-aortic balloon counterpulsation, surgery as last resort

**Complications:** Acute, severe mitral regurgitation

## 1.42  VALVULAR DISEASES: TRICUSPID REGURGITATION

**Etiology:** Secondary to a combination of dilation and high pressure due to severe pulmonary HTN or outflow obstruction, RV and inferior MI, SLE, IVDA endocarditis

**S/S:**
- Sensation of pulsations in neck, atrial fib or flutter, hepatomegaly, JVD, dyspnea, ascites, systolic thrill at L lower SB, +/− pulsatile liver
- Murmur—harsh, blowing, systolic, along lower L sternal border, CARVALLO'S SIGN

**Dx:**
- ECG—RV overload
- CXR—enlargement of superior vena cava and R atrium, +/− RV enlargement
- Echo—evaluates valvular apparatus and cavity size; Doppler jet evaluation of the regurgitant valve and R-sided heart pressures

**Tx:** Treat heart failure as needed; valve repair or valvuloplasty; replacement as a last resort

**Complications:** R-sided heart failure

## 1.43  VALVULAR DISEASES: TRICUSPID STENOSIS

**Etiology:** Rheumatic heart disease, always accompanies mitral stenosis

**S/S:**
- Fatigue, fluttering discomfort in the neck (caused by giant A wave in jugular pulse), hepatomegaly, ascites, dependent edema, "olive" color of skin (mixed jaundice and cyanosis)
- Murmur—diastolic rumbling along lower L sternal border

**Dx:**
- ECG—tall, peaked P waves in inferior leads and $V_1$
- CXR—dilated R atrium and superior vena cava
- Echo—tricuspid thickening, ↓ early diastolic filling slope of tricuspid valve

**Tx:** Symptomatic treatment, rarely requires valve replacement

**Complications:** R-sided heart failure

Takayasu's arteritis

Granulomatous vasculitis c̄ intimal fibrosis & vascular narrowing

Mc affects aorta & pulmonary arteries

MC in young or middle-aged women of Asian descent

Leads to massive intimal fibrosis → arterial stenosis, thrombosis, & aneurysms

Dx: MR angiography, CT angiography, arterial angiography (DSA)

S/SXS: "Inflammatory phase" → malaise, fever, night sweats, weight loss, arthralgia, & fatigue

"Pulseless phase" → vascular insufficiency → claudication, renal artery stenosis & HTN, brain hypoperfusion & lightheadedness & seizures, visual field defects

late → localized aneurysms, Raynaud's phenomenon

TX: low-dose corticosteroids, percutaneous transluminal coronary angioplasty (PTCA), bypass grafting

# CHAPTER 2

# Pulmonary System

## 2.1 ADULT RESPIRATORY DISTRESS SYNDROME

**Etiology:** Lung injury, either direct (pneumonia, aspiration of GI contents, pulmonary contusion, fat emboli, drowning, toxic inhalation) or indirect (sepsis, trauma, shock, transfusions, pancreatitis, drugs), leads to generalized lung inflammation → ↑ pulmonary vascular permeability, interstitial edema, alveolar consolidation, and atelectasis

**S/S:** Rapid onset of profound dyspnea, labored breathing, tachypnea, IC retractions, rales, severe hypoxemia with poor response to supplemental oxygen, extreme V/Q mismatch, diffuse crackles, rhonchi, rapid respiratory failure; usually requires mechanical ventilation with high peak airway pressures

**Dx:** Three criteria for diagnosis:
1. CXR—diffuse or patchy B/L infiltrates, sparing the costophrenic angle
2. Blood gas or pulse oximetry—hypoxemia
3. Absence of cardiogenic pulmonary edema

**Tx:**
- ID and treat underlying cause
- Aggressive supportive care
- Ventilator management—(1) permissive hypercapnia (small tidal volumes to prevent overstretching of healthy alveoli; (2) avoid oxygen toxicity, ↑ PEEP, not $FiO_2$
- Glucocorticoids may be used but must not be started **before** day 7 (starting early ↑ morbidity)

**Complications:** Death, fibrotic lung injury, pulmonary hypertension

## 2.2 ASBESTOS PNEUMOCONIOSIS

**Etiology:** Inflammation and fibrosis due to inhalation of asbestos fibers; results in progressive lung fibrosis that may progress even without continued exposure

**S/S:** Gradual, progressive dyspnea, nonproductive cough, hypoxemia, tachypnea, crackles, clubbing, decreased lung volume, end stage = right-sided heart failure, cor pulmonale

**Dx:**
- History of exposure
- PFTs—restrictive pattern with decreased lung volumes
- CXR—irregular linear opacities, pleural thickening, calcific pleural plaques, +/− pleural effusion, ground-glass infiltrate
- CT—subpleural curvilinear lines parallel to pleural surface, fibrosis

**Tx:** Avoid further exposure, no smoking, supplemental oxygen if needed

**Complications:** Increased risk of bronchogenic carcinoma and malignant mesothelioma, death due to respiratory failure or cancer

## 2.3  ASTHMA

**Etiology:** Chronic inflammation characterized by 3 elements:
1. Chronic airway inflammation
2. Bronchial hyperreactivity
3. Reversible airway obstruction

**S/S:**
- Cough, dyspnea/SOB, tightness in chest, expiratory wheezing, sleep disturbances
- Mild attack—slight tachycardia, tachypnea, diffuse wheezing with prolonged expirations
- Severe attack—accessory muscle use, intercostal retractions, hyperresonance, distant breath sounds
- Late severe—fatigue, diaphoresis, decreased breath sounds/wheezing, cyanosis, PULSUS PARADOXUS

**Dx:**
- PFT—↓ FEV, ↑ TLC, ↑ RV
- CXR—hyperinflation, +/− atelectasis
- ABG—respiratory alkalosis, hypoxemia, metabolic acidosis
- Sputum culture—↑ eosinophils

**Tx:**
- Avoid triggers, give supplemental oxygen if needed
- Medications—bronchodilators, inhaled corticosteroids, anticholinergics
- Severe attacks—systemic steroids, nebulized bronchodilators, +/− theophylline

**Complications:** exhaustion, dehydration, airway infection, tussive syncope, STATUS ASTHMATICUS, cor pulmonale

## 2.4  ASTHMA, SPECIFIC TYPES

**Exercise-Induced Asthma:** Occurs only in patients with a known history of asthma; attack occurs 5–10 min after starting to exercise

**Triad Asthma:** Combination of intrinsic asthma, aspirin sensitivity, and nasal polyposis; occurs in < 10% of asthma patients

**Occupational Asthma:** Triggered by various agents found in the workplace; may occur weeks to years after initial exposure

**Cardiac Asthma:** Bronchospasm precipitated by CHF

**Drug-Induced Asthma:** Caused by many common medications (aspirin, propranolol, NSAIDs, beta blockers, histamine, methacholine, any nebulized medicine)

**Asthmatic Bronchitis:** Chronic bronchitis with features of bronchospasm that quickly responds to bronchodilator therapy

## 2.5 BRONCHIECTASIS

**Definition:** Abnormal, irreversible dilation of the medium-sized airways

**Etiology:** Inflammatory insult (usually infectious) leads to fibrosis, which causes dilated and distorted airways that cannot properly clear secretions; cystic fibrosis causes approximately 50% of all cases

**S/S:**
- Classic triad—persistent productive cough, copious purulent sputum, hemoptysis
- Recurrent pneumonia, dyspnea, crackles, rhonchi, wheezing, fever, weight loss, anemia, pleuritic CP, clubbing, pulmonary hypertension, cor pulmonale

**Dx:**
- CT—dilated airways, "TRAM TRACKS" parallel to each other, "SIGNET RING" BRONCHIOLES
- CXR—may be normal; if abnormal, cystic areas with fluid levels, peribronchial thickening, "TRAM TRACKS," and atelectasis may be seen
- Sputum Cx—neutrophils
- Sweat chloride—to evaluate for cystic fibrosis (presents in adulthood in 4% of cases)
- PFTs—determine if restrictive or mixed restrictive-obstructive disorder

**Tx:** Treat underlying cause; improve clearance of secretions (bronchodilators, postural drainage, chest PT); control infections; surgical resections (for localized disease only); lung transplants

**Complications:** Respiratory failure, recurrent respiratory infections

## 2.6 BRONCHIOLITIS

**Etiology:** Usually secondary to viral infection (RSV, parainfluenza, influenza, and adenovirus); causes inflammatory obstruction of the peripheral airways

**Risk Factors:** Children who were born prematurely or with chronic lung disease, congenital heart disease, and congenital or acquired immunodeficiency are more susceptible to severe disease

**S/S:** Fever, cough, rhinorrhea, followed by progressive respiratory distress, tachypnea, wheezing, rhonchi, crackles, accessory muscle use, hypoxia in severe cases

**Dx:** CXR—diffuse nonspecific alveolar or "ground-glass" densities

**Tx:** Oral systemic steroids, supportive respiratory care; severe cases require hospitalization with supplemental oxygen

**Complications:** Apnea (neonates), relapse, BOOP (bronchiolitis obliterans organizing pneumonia)

## 2.7  BRONCHITIS, ACUTE

**Etiology:** Viruses or *Mycoplasma pneumoniae*

**S/S:** General malaise, fever/chills, myalgias, +/− sore throat, cough (nonproductive early, progressing to mucopurulent sputum), substernal discomfort (worse with coughing), scattered high- or low-pitched rhonchi, crackles or moist rales at the bases, wheezing

**Dx:**
- CXR—normal
- Sputum C&S—indicated for nonresponsive cases

**Tx:** Symptomatic, antibiotics if needed for a secondary infection (pneumonia, pharyngitis, sinusitis)

**Complications:** Pneumonia, pharyngitis, sinusitis, acute respiratory failure

## 2.8  BRONCHITIS, CHRONIC (TYPE B COPD)

**Etiology:** Excessive secretion of bronchial mucus with a productive cough for 3 months or more in at least 2 consecutive years with no other disease that might account for these symptoms

**S/S:** "Blue bloater"—productive cough, exertional dyspnea, fatigue, rhonchi/wheezing, central cyanosis, hypoxia, often obese habitus, plethora

**Dx:**
- CXR—increased markings ("dirty lungs"), large horizontal heart, localized fibrosis or bronchiectasis
- PFTs—obstructive pattern ($\downarrow$ FEV$_1$/FVC)
- ABG—hypoxemia, hypercarbia
- CBC—polycythemia
- ECG—R axis deviation, RVH

**Tx:** no smoking, bronchodilators, supplemental oxygen, chest PT, +/− steroids

**Complications:** Pulmonary hypertension, cor pulmonale, chronic respiratory failure, LVF

## 2.9 BRONCHOGENIC CARCINOMA

**Etiology:** Five types:

1. Squamous cell carcinoma—originates in central bronchi as intraluminal growth, early mets to regional lymph nodes
2. Adenocarcinoma—appears in the periphery, early mets to distant organs
3. Bronchoalveolar cell carcinoma—specific type of adenocarcinoma, low grade, presents as single or multiple nodules or as alveolar infiltrate
4. Small cell carcinoma—"oat cell" occurs centrally, very early widespread mets (100% in smokers)
5. Large cell carcinoma—occurs at periphery, often cavitary lesions, early mets

**S/S:** Cough, weight loss, dyspnea, CP, hemoptysis, atelectasis, postobstructive pneumonitis, pleural effusion, lymphadenopathy, hepatomegaly, clubbing

**Dx:**
- Cytology exam of sputum to get tissue diagnosis
- CXR—some type of abnormality, depending on type of carcinoma, usually found

**Tx:** Chemotherapy, radiation therapy, surgical resection—any combination or all

**Complications:** Mets, recurrence, death (5-year survival is between 10 and 15%)

## 2.10 CYSTIC FIBROSIS

**Etiology:**
- Defect in the cystic fibrosis transmembrane receptor protein; affects various organ systems
- Presents in adulthood in 4% of cases
- Lungs—abnormal sodium transport causes thick, poorly cleared mucus, resulting in chronic bacterial colonization and recurrent infections
- Pancreas—thickened secretions result in retention of pancreatic enzymes, with steatorrhea and eventual destruction of the pancreas

**S/S:**
- Pulmonary—chronic cough, purulent sputum, wheezing, SOB, chronic sinusitis, clubbing, nasal polyps, hemoptysis, pneumothorax, recurrent infections and pneumonia
- GI—pancreatic insufficiency, protein/fat malabsorption, diabetes, obstruction/intussusception, biliary stasis, constipation, sterility

**Dx:**
- Sweat chloride test is diagnostic
- PFT—obstructive pattern ($\downarrow$ FVC, $\uparrow$ lung volume)
- CXR—hyperinflation, peribronchial cuffing, bronchiectasis
- ABG—hypoxemia, metabolic alkalosis
- Electrolytes—hypochloremia, hyponatremia, metabolic alkalosis, hyperglycemia

**Tx:** Inhaled antibiotics ($\uparrow$ lung function and $\downarrow$ exacerbations), chest PT, bronchodilators, high-fat diet, vitamin supplements, control airway inflammation, lung transplant

**Complications:** Chronic course with acute exacerbations, respiratory failure major cause of death

## 2.11 EMPHYSEMA (TYPE A COPD)

**Definition:** Abnormal, permanent enlargement of airspaces distal to the terminal bronchiole, with destruction of their walls and without obvious fibrosis

**Etiology:** Smoking (most cases), genetic predisposition, air pollution, occupational exposure to irritants, allergy

**S/S:** "Pink puffers"—severe dyspnea, hypertrophy of accessory muscles, increased AP chest diameter, hyperresonance, minimal to no cough, decreased air movement, "tripod" position, decreased breath sounds, weight loss

**Dx:**
- CXR—bullae, blebs, decreased markings in periphery, hyperinflation with low, flat hemidiaphragm
- ABG—normal $P_{CO_2}$, minimal hypoxemia
- PFTs—↑ TLC, ↓ diffusing capacity

**Tx:** No smoking, bronchodilators, supplemental $O_2$ if needed, theophylline, lung volume reduction surgery or lung transplant for end-stage disease

**Complications:** Acute exacerbations, infections, pulmonary hypertension, cor pulmonale, progression to respiratory failure

## 2.12 EPIGLOTTITIS

**Etiology:** Inflammation and edema of the epiglottis and aryepiglottic folds secondary to infection; most common pathogens: *Strep. pneumoniae*, group A streptococcus, *Haemophilus influenzae*

**S/S:** Fever, sore throat, hoarseness, stridor, severe respiratory distress; child presents leaning forward with chin extended, with moderate drooling

**Dx:**
- Lateral neck x-ray—"thumbprinting" of epiglottis
- Throat and blood Cx—culture throat in OR only after airway is secure; C&S needed to direct treatment

**Tx:**
- Emergent endotracheal intubation; if unable to secure airway, proceed immediately to cricothyroidotomy
- IV ampicillin/sulbactam empirically until cultures return
- IV hydration and aggressive pulmonary toilet to maintain airway patency imperative until airway is stabilized

**Complications:** Airway obstruction, death

## 2.13 OBSTRUCTIVE SLEEP APNEA

**Etiology:** Upper airway soft tissue impedes airflow

**Risk Factors:** Narrow airway (obesity, macroglossia), ETOH, sedatives, smoking, vocal cord dysfunction, bulbar disease

**S/S:** Loud snoring, restlessness or thrashing during sleep, obesity, narrowed oropharynx, daytime somnolence and fatigue, morning sluggishness, cognitive impairment, HA

**Dx:**
- Overnight polysomnography is diagnostic
- CBC—erythrocytosis

**Tx:** Avoid ETOH and sedatives, weight reduction, oral dental prosthesis, nasal septoplasty, CPAP, bypass tracheostomy in life-threatened patients

**Complications:** Cardiac arrhythmias, pulmonary hypertension, cor pulmonale, CHF, hypertension, erythrocytosis

## 2.14 PLEURISY

**Etiology:** Pleural injury secondary to pneumonia, infarction; entry of an infectious agent or irritant (amebic empyema, pancreatitic pleurisy); neoplastic metastases; TB; RA; SLE; pleural trauma; asbestos-related pleural disease

**S/S:** Fever/chills; localized, sharp, fleeting pain that increases with cough, sneeze, or deep breathing; +/− radiation of pain to shoulder; shallow, rapid breathing

**Dx:** Clinical diagnosis; +/− pleural friction rub

**Tx:** Treat any underlying disease; analgesics, anti-inflammatories, codeine cough suppressants; encourage pulmonary toilet

**Complications:** Pneumonia

## 2.15 PNEUMONIA

**Etiology:** Lower respiratory tract infection of lung parenchyma, results in inflammation, alveolar exudates, and consolidation

**S/S:** Fever, dyspnea, productive cough, rigors, sweats, chills, chest discomfort, fatigue, myalgias, anorexia, HA, abdominal pain, N/V, tachypnea, dullness to percussion, tachycardia, <u>EGOPHONY</u>, hypoxemia, rhonchi

**Dx:**
- Pulse oximetry
- CXR—from patchy infiltrates to consolidation
- Sputum Cx—identifies causative pathogen
- Blood Cx—for all hospitalized patients (rule out sepsis)

**Tx:**
- Antibiotics specific to the pathogen if identified
- CAP—macrolide, doxycycline, or quinolone
- For hospitalized patients, add cephalosporin (2nd or 3rd generation)
- HAP—3rd-generation cephalosporin or beta-lactam/beta-lactamase inhibitor

*Macrolides: Azithromycin, Clarithromycin*
*Quinolones: Ciprofloxacin, Levofloxacin*

**Complications:** Respiratory failure, sepsis, death

## 2.16 PNEUMONIA, SPECIFIC TYPES

**Types:**
- Acute bacterial pneumonia (bact)
- Atypical pneumonia (atypic)
- Anaerobic pneumonia (anaerob)

**Etiology:**
- Bact—*Strep. pneumoniae* or *Pseudomonas* (nosocomial)
- Atypic—*Mycoplasma pneumoniae*
- Anaerob—usually secondary to aspiration, includes all anaerobes in oral flora

**S/S:**
- Bact—acute onset fever/chills, purulent sputum
- Atypic—fever, malaise, HA, nonproductive cough
- Anaerob—fever, weight loss, malaise, foul-smelling, purulent sputum

**Dx:**
- Labs: Bact—↑ WBC with L shift; sputum = neutrophils, a single predominant organism; Atypic—leukocytosis; sputum = neutrophils, mononuclear cells, no predominant organism; Anaerob—obtain sample to culture via transtracheal or thoracic aspiration
- CXR: Bact—lobar or segmental infiltrates; Atypic—patchy, nonlobar infiltrates; Anaerob—lung abscess or empyema

**Tx:**
- Bact—healthy patient without complications: treat as outpatient with oral antibiotics; mild to severe cases require inpatient treatment with bed rest, supplemental oxygen as needed, antibiotics, chest PT
- Atypic—erythromycin
- Anaerobic—PCN G, clindamycin; drainage of any pleural fluid or abscess is mandatory

## 2.17 PNEUMOTHORAX

**Etiology:** Trauma, iatrogenic
- Spontaneous—primary = no underlying lung disease; secondary = coexisting lung disease (COPD, asthma, CF, infection, CA, interstitial)
- Tension—occurs when a check-valve mechanism permits air to enter but not leave the pleural space

**S/S:**
- Acute pleuritic CP, dyspnea, tachypnea, tachycardia, decreased breath sounds on affected side, hyperresonance to percussion, decreased TACTILE FREMITUS, +/− respiratory distress
- Tension—hypotension, absent breath sounds, distended jugular veins, tracheal deviation, diaphoresis, cyanosis, cardiovascular collapse

**Dx:**
- CXR—presence of thin radiolucent pleural line, absence of vascular lung markings peripheral to pleural line, tracheal deviation to opposite side of pneumothorax (tension)
- ECG—tachycardia, nonspecific ST-segment changes, T-wave inversion
- ABG—hypoxia, normal $P_{CO_2}$

**Tx:** 100% oxygen, emergent needle thoracotomy (tension), chest tube placement

**Complications:** Recurrence, death

## 2.18 PULMONARY EMBOLISM

**Etiology:** Clot from DVT in LE or R side of heart, fat embolus, air embolus, amniotic fluid embolus

**Risk Factors:** LE venous disease, CA, CHF, recent surgery, immobilization, family history, pregnancy/childbirth, paraplegia, previous DVT, OCP, trauma, hypercoagulable state, advanced age

**S/S:** Dyspnea, pleuritic CP, tachypnea, tachycardia, anxiety, cough, crackles, +/− fevers, hemoptysis, evidence of LE DVT (swelling, + HOMANS' SIGN), syncope, hypotension, R-sided HF

**Dx:**
- Pulmonary angio—"gold standard"
- V/Q scan—normal scan rules out PE, but any mismatch requires further workup
- Spiral CT—sensitive for proximal PE, distal PE sensitivity uncertain, good noninvasive screening
- D-Dimer—nonspecific test confirms hypercoagulability; does not identify PE, only those at risk
- Doppler US—good noninvasive screening test for those at risk, not specific (negative test does not rule out PE)

**Tx:**
- Supportive—supplemental oxygen, IV fluid, pressors as needed
- Anticoagulation—heparin, low-molecular-weight heparin, warfarin
- Thrombolytic therapy—for acute PE only
- Thrombolectomy via angiogram or open
- Vena cava filter for those at risk who are not candidates for anticoagulation

**Complications:** Lung infarction, recurrent PE, death

## 2.19 PULMONARY TUBERCULOSIS

**Etiology:** *Mycobacterium tuberculosis*

**S/S:** Fatigue, weight loss, anorexia, low-grade fever, night sweats, cough (starts off dry, progresses to productive with purulent or bloody sputum), posttussive apical rales

**Dx:**
- CXR—upper lobe/apical infiltrates (small, homogeneous), hilar and paratracheal lymph node enlargement, segmental atelectasis, +/− pleural effusion
- Labs—sputum culture: must obtain sample, if patient unable to produce sputum requires bronchoscopy with bronchial washing

**Tx: All cases must be reported to local and state public health departments**
- Active TB—respiratory isolation, isoniazid and rifampin for 6 months plus pyrazinamide for 2 months; add ethambutol in areas of isoniazid resistance (most of USA) pending sensitivities
- Latent TB—isoniazid for 9 months OR rifampin for 4 months; if isoniazid-resistant, use rifampin and pyrazinamide for 2 months

**Complications:** Spontaneous pneumothorax, cavity formation and marked fibrosis, respiratory failure, pulmonary hypertension, cor pulmonale, seeding of extrapulmonary areas

## 2.20 SARCOIDOSIS

**Etiology:** A systemic, granulomatous, inflammatory disorder of unknown cause; predominantly affects lungs, but 50% have other systems involved (with or without lungs involved)

**S/S:** Cough, dyspnea, chest discomfort, hemoptysis, fever, weight loss, fatigue, polyarthritis, uveitis; neurologic, cardiac, dermatologic, hepatic systems may also be affected

**Dx:**
- Diagnosis of exclusion, confirmed by biopsy showing noncaseating granulomas: sample from lymph node, bronchi, skin lesion, salivary glands, liver
- CXR—bilateral hilar lymphadenopathy
- CT—nonspecific alveolitis; diffuse nodular adenopathy
- ECG—conduction disorders (if cardiac involvement)

**Tx:**
- Observation for 6 months recommended for isolated pulmonary involvement; most will remit spontaneously
- Severe or progressive or with extrapulmonary involvement; systemic steroids = the mainstay
- Bronchodilators for symptomatic relief
- Lung transplant for life-threatening cases

**Complications:** Recurrence (even after lung transplant); irreversible lung fibrosis, bronchiectasis, respiratory failure

## 2.21 SOLITARY PULMONARY NODULE

**Etiology:** 60% are benign (infectious granulomas), 40% malignant (primary lung CA)

**S/S:** Depends on site and location; most are asymptomatic and are an incidental finding on CXR

**Dx:** CXR: round/oval sharply circumscribed pulmonary lesion (<5 cm) surrounded by normal lung tissue

**Tx:** All should be considered malignant and be resected unless calcification on CXR typical of benign lesions is noted or stability on CXR is documented for at least 2 years

**Complications:** 25% of all bronchogenic carcinoma present as solitary lesions; 50% five-year survival rate if detected and treated at this early stage

CHAPTER 3

# Gastrointestinal System and Nutrition

## 3.1 ACHALASIA: MEDICAL PERSPECTIVE

**Etiology:** Major dysfunction of esophageal smooth muscle peristalsis and abnormal LES tone ($\uparrow$ LES resting pressure and failure of LES to relax in response to swallowing)

**S/S:** Progressive dysphagia, vomiting of food a few hours after eating, weight loss, nocturnal cough (due to aspiration), chest pain, heartburn, bloating, inability to burp, aspiration, and respiratory infections

**Dx:**
- X-ray—dilated esophagus, "bird beak" narrowing at LES, widening of mediastinum, air-fluid level in esophagus
- Manometer—LES = $\uparrow$ resting pressure and incomplete relaxation with swallowing; body = failure of peristalsis; low-amplitude, abnormal, or absent contractions after swallowing
- Endoscopy—obtain biopsy to rule out neoplasia

**Tx:**
- Palliative—nitrates and calcium channel blockers; forced dilation of LES with pneumatic bag; botulinum toxin injection (only if unable to dilate)
- Surgical—esophagomyotomy (high risk for postoperative GERD)

**Complications:** Tenfold increased risk of esophageal cancer, recurrence (with dilation), GERD (with surgery)

## 3.2 ACUTE ABDOMEN

**Etiology:**
- Surgical—perforated peptic ulcer, acute cholecystitis, acute/chronic pancreatitis, acute appendicitis, PID, ovarian cysts, ectopic pregnancy, renal calculi, Meckel's diverticulum, acute diverticulitis, acute small bowel obstruction, acute large bowl obstruction, volvulus
- Nonsurgical—pneumonia, MI, DKA, hepatitis, musculoskeletal pain

**S/S:** Pain—type, quality, and location depend on etiology; bowel habit changes; menstrual changes or pain associated with menses

**Dx:**
- Labs—CBC, chem panel, LFT, UA, amylase, beta hCG
- Supine and upright x-ray of abdomen
- US +/− CT or arteriography

**Indications for Surgery:** Acute abdominal pain > 6 hr, abdominal rigidity, increased or localized pain with palpation, progressive abdominal distention, abdominal pain associated with shock/septicemia, labs indicating gut ischemia ($\uparrow$ lactate, metabolic acidosis), declining VS or ms, pneumoperitoneum, bowel or cecal distention, extravasation of contrast on enema or SBFT, mesenteric artery occlusion, intra-abdominal hemorrhage

## 3.3  ALCOHOLIC LIVER DISEASE

**Etiology:** Excess alcohol intake over many years, 2 stages:

1. Acute—fatty liver and alcoholic hepatitis, reversible with abstinence
2. Chronic—cirrhosis, irreversible

**S/S:**
- Fatty liver—asymptomatic hepatomegaly
- Chronic = s/s of <u>HEPATITIS</u>, <u>CIRRHOSIS</u>, <u>ACUTE</u> <u>PANCREATITIS</u>, <u>CHRONIC</u> <u>PANCREATITIS</u>
- Spider angiomas, ascites, encephalopathy

**Dx:** Labs—↑ liver enzymes with AST:ALT ratio 2:1; AST < 400; ↑ alkaline phosphatase; ↑ bilirubin; hypoalbuminemia; biopsy is diagnostic

**Tx:**
- Early recognition and treatment of alcoholism are paramount
- 4-week course oral prednisone for alcoholic hepatitis or hepatic encephalopathy
- Thiamine, folate, and vitamin $B_{12}$ supplementation

**Complications:** Cirrhosis, hepatic failure, GI hemorrhage, infection, hepatorenal syndrome, hepatocellular carcinoma

## 3.4  ANAL FISSURE

**Etiology:** A linear disruption of the anal epithelium due to various causes

**S/S:**
- Acute pain during and after defecation
- Spotting of bright red blood on stool
- Tendency toward constipation
- Late occurrence of a sentinel pile
- Hypertrophied papilla
- Spasm of the anal canal

**Dx:** Clinical diagnosis

**Tx:**
- Regulation of bowel habits with use of bulking agent +/− stool softeners
- Sitz baths
- +/− suppositories bid
- Surgical excision for refractory cases

**Complications:** Infection, sentinel pile

## 3.5 BOWEL OBSTRUCTION

**Etiology:**
- Small—adhesions, hernia, tumor
- Large—colon CA, volvulus, diverticulitis
- May be acute/chronic; partial/complete; mechanical (adhesions/hernia) or paralytic/impaired motility (trauma, surgery, hypokalemia, peritonitis); simple/strangulated (cuts off vascular supply)

**S/S:**
- Crampy, intermittent abdominal pain, distention, vomiting, constipation
- Mechanical obstruction—high-pitched BS with peristaltic rushes and tinkles
- Ileus—decreased or absent BS

**Dx:**
- Flat and upright ABD x-ray—excess air in small bowel, no air in colon; air-fluid level in distended loops of bowel, normal bowel distal to obstruction; diffuse gas if ileus, leukocytosis (strangulated bowel)
- Enema with Gastrografin solution to diagnose obstruction

**Tx:** IV fluids, NG suction, correct electrolyte abnormalities, monitor urine output, treat underlying causes

**Indications for Surgery:** Strangulated bowel, complete obstruction, partial obstruction with worsening course

**Complications:** Strangulated bowel—necrosis and gangrene, sepsis, death

## 3.6 CIRRHOSIS

**Definition:** Irreversible destruction of liver architecture by nodules of fibrosis

**Etiology:** Chronic alcohol abuse, viral hepatitis, any chronic liver disease, massive acute injury

**S/S:** Firm, nodular liver, ascites, hepatosplenomegaly, CAPUT MEDUSA, esophageal varices, jaundice, spider angioma, palmar erythema, gynecomastia, testicular atrophy, bruising, hypocoagulopathies, hepatic encephalopathy

**Dx:**
- US or ABD CT
- Biopsy is diagnostic
- Labs—liver enzymes ↑ early, ↓ when significant cirrhosis ensues; hypoalbuminemia; hypocholesterolemia; electrolyte disturbances; azotemia; ↑ PTT

**Tx:** Treat underlying liver disease, avoid alcohol, stabilize electrolytes, low-protein diet, lactulose

**Complications:** Portal hypertension, esophageal varices, encephalopathy, ascites

## 3.7  CIRRHOSIS, PRIMARY BILIARY

**Etiology:** Chronic disease of cholestasis due to granulomatous destruction of intrahepatic bile ducts; most likely of immunologic cause

**S/S:** Pruritus and persistent fatigue, evidence of advanced liver disease (jaundice and ascites), hepatosplenomegaly, steatorrhea

**Dx:**
- Labs—↑ alkaline phosphatase and bilirubin; + AMA antibodies in > 90% of patients; + ANA in some patients; transaminases normal or slightly elevated (< 200)
- Biopsy is diagnostic
- US or ERCP may be used

**Tx:** Ursodeoxycholic acid may be effective; liver transplant is curative

**Complications:** Cirrhosis, osteoporosis, deficiency of fat-soluble vitamins (A, D, E, K), hypercholesterolemia, malabsorption, renal tubular necrosis

## 3.8  COLON CARCINOMA

**Etiology:** 98% are adenocarcinomas, almost always arising from adenomatous polyps

**S/S:**
- Change in bowel habits; ↓ stool size; fatigue, weakness; weight loss; abdominal discomfort; inguinal lymphadenopathy
- Obstruction—N/V, fever, tachycardia, no BM or flatus
- R-sided—postprandial discomfort, +/– R-sided mass, iron deficiency anemia
- L-sided—alternating diarrhea and constipation, hematochezia, +/– L-sided mass, ↑ risk of obstruction
- Rectal—tenesmus, mass on digital rectal exam (DRE)

**Dx:**
- Screening—annual DRE, stool guaiac, sigmoidoscopy every 3–5 yr after age 50
- BE—evaluate for polyps
- Colonoscopy is diagnostic
- CEA—not good for screening, useful to evaluate for recurrence or mets
- CXR, LFTs, alkaline phosphatase, RFT to evaluate for mets

**Tx:** Surgery—curative early (Duke A & B); surgery plus chemotherapy—Duke C; surgery for palliation—Duke D; radiation treatment preoperatively for rectal lesions

**Complications:** Mets, recurrence, death

## 3.9 CROHN'S DISEASE

**Etiology:** Chronic granulomatous disease; may affect any part of the GI tract, primarily ileum; characterized by <u>SKIP</u> <u>LESIONS</u> with full thickness of colonic wall involved

**S/S:** Colicky abdominal pain, fever, weight loss, anal disease, +/− steatorrhea, occult blood, melena, diarrhea, RLQ mass (extensive ileal involvement), enteropathic arthropathy (10%)

**Dx:**
- ABD x-ray
- Endoscopy—inflammatory changes, rectal sparing, skip lesions
- Biopsy—inflammation, granulomas
- Small bowel follow-through: "<u>STRING</u> <u>SIGN</u>"

**Tx:**
- Daily—sulfasalazine, 5-ASA, mesalamine
- Flare-ups—bowel rest (NPO, NGT), IV fluids, TPN, steroids, antibiotics
- Surgery—only for severe disease or complications

**Complications:** Perforation, fistula to other organs, abscess, obstruction, adhesions, recurrence, nephrolithiasis, hypocalcemia, vitamin $B_{12}$ deficiency, strictures, increased risk for colon CA

## 3.10 DIVERTICULAR DISEASE

**Types:**
- Diverticulosis (sis)
- Diverticulitis (tis)
- Diverticular bleeding (bld)

**Etiology:**
- sis—asymptomatic outpouching of colon
- tis—infection and inflammation of a diverticulum
- bld—most common cause of lower GI bleeding in the elderly

**S/S:**
- sis—usually asymptomatic; may have lower abdominal pain relieved by BM, alternating diarrhea and constipation
- tis—LLQ pain ↑ with BM, +/− mass LLQ, tenderness to palpation over LLQ (rebound tenderness indicates perforation)
- bld—painless rectal bleeding, +/− hematochezia, shock

**Dx:**
- CT is diagnostic
- ABD x-ray—diverticula look like "thumbprints" along colon
- Upright ABD x-ray—free air under diaphragm if perforated

**Tx:**
- sis—high-fiber diet
- tis—bowel rest, broad-spectrum antibiotics, percutaneous drainage of abscess if needed, colonic resection after 2nd bout (recommended after 1st bout in young patients)
- bld—stabilize patient, identify source of bleeding, sigmoidectomy if intractable bleeding

**Complications:** Colon CA, recurrence, perforation, adhesions, sepsis, death

## 3.11 ESOPHAGEAL CARCINOMA

**Types:**
- Squamous cell (S)
- Adenocarcinoma (A)
- Barrett's esophagitis (B)

**Etiology:**
- S—dietary and environmental factors (tobacco, ETOH, vitamins A and C deficiency)
- A—GERD, Barrett's esophagitis
- B—columnar epithelium replaces the normal squamous epithelium of the distal esophagus following chronic inflammation secondary to GERD

**S/S:** Progressive dysphagia for solids, extreme weight loss, cough, hoarseness, choking and aspiration pneumonia due to tracheoesophageal fistula, bleeding, chest pain, vomiting

**Dx:** Barium swallow if obstruction suspected; endoscopy with biopsy is diagnostic

**Tx:**
- Surgical resection for lower-third lesions; recurrence is common
- Radiation +/– chemotherapy for S; A does not respond well to radiation therapy
- Laser therapy for intraluminal tumors

**Complications:** Strictures, obstruction, metastases, recurrence

## 3.12 ESOPHAGEAL VARICES

**Etiology:** Prolonged or severe portal hypertension

**S/S:**
- Asymptomatic until rupture
- Rupture—painless but massive hematemesis of dark-brown blood; pallor, tachycardia, orthostasis, physical signs of cirrhosis of the liver (hepatomegaly, splenomegaly, ascites, jaundice, palmar erythema, clubbing, spider angiomas, parotid enlargement, bitemporal wasting)

**Dx:** Endoscopy—should be done as soon as patient is hemodynamically stable

**Tx:**
- Supportive—volume replacement, FFP, close monitoring of hemodynamic status, airway control
- Endoscopy to identify and treat the bleeding with sclerotherapy and/or banding
- Balloon tamponade may be used if endoscopy unavailable or bleeding persists after endoscopy
- IV octreotide or vasopressin
- Emergent surgery if bleeding persists

**Complications:** Recurrence, shock, death

## 3.13 ESOPHAGITIS

**Etiology:** Inflammation of the esophageal mucosa following injury or infection

**Risk Factors:** GERD; infection (*Candida*, HSV, CMV, HIV), chemical irritants (ETOH, cigarette smoke, very hot fluids, alkali, acids, drugs)

**S/S:** Heartburn, dysphagia (solids > liquids), odynophagia, anemia

**Dx:** History of caustic ingestion or immunosuppression is red flag, endoscopy, esophagoscopy, manometry or acid reflux test

**Tx:**
- Reflux—treat as GERD
- Infectious—use appropriate antimicrobial
- Irritants—broad-spectrum antibiotics and steroids

**Complications:** Stricture formation (due to chronic inflammation and fibrosis), esophageal ulceration with possible hemorrhage, efflux laryngitis, pulmonary aspiration, Barrett's esophagus

## 3.14 GASTRIC CARCINOMA

**Etiology:** 95% are adenocarcinoma; 2 primary types of tumors:
1. Intestinal—most common type, grows as a cohesive tumor and eventually erodes through the stomach wall to nearby organs
2. Diffuse—a poorly differentiated tumor that has little cell cohesion, it grows outward along the submucosa of the stomach and widely envelopes the stomach without producing a discrete mass

**S/S:** Epigastric pain, postprandial fullness, anorexia, nausea, weight loss, vomiting (if pyloric tumor), dysphagia (if cardia tumor), occult hemorrhage, palpable ABD mass (advanced tumors)

**Dx:**
- Double-contrast barium enema, endoscopy with biopsy is diagnostic
- ABD CT
- CXR +/− CT chest
- Labs—CBC, LFTs

**Tx:** Surgery is the only potential cure
- Total gastrectomy (proximal lesion); subtotal gastrectomy (distal lesion)
- Lymphadenectomy is important and varies in extent based on stage and physician preference
- Resection of adjacent organs depends on the level of involvement
- Radiation and/or chemotherapy useful as palliative treatment for symptoms

**Complications:** Metastases, perforation, obstruction

## 3.15 GASTRITIS

**Types:**
- Acute erosive gastritis (A)
- Chronic gastritis (C)

**Etiology:**
- A—self-limited irritation of mucosa due to NSAIDs, ETOH, or severe physiologic stress (major surgery, burns, ventilator)
- C—type A, less common, involves proximal stomach only, due to pernicious anemia, atrophic gastritis, autoimmune disease, radiation; type B, most common, involves distal stomach and antrum, due to *Helicobacter pylori* infection

**S/S:** Burning epigastric pain, dyspepsia, N/V, hematemesis, shock, microcytic anemia (C)

**Dx:**
- Endoscopy is diagnostic
- *H. pylori* testing—serologic tests, biopsy, culture
- Labs—CBC, Schilling test

**Tx:** Manage hemodynamic instability in hemorrhage; avoid offending agents; H$_2$ blockers, antacids, sucralfate; *H. pylori*—treat only if symptomatic, 10- to 14-day course with triple therapy (never monotherapy)

**Complications:** Gastric ulcers, gastric cancer

## 3.16 GASTROESOPHAGEAL REFLUX DISEASE

**Etiology:** Characterized by incompetence of lower esophageal sphincter (LES), irregular peristalsis, altered mucosal resistance, and abnormally slow gastric emptying; associated with recently ingested fat in duodenum, full stomach, smoking, pregnancy, supine position, caffeine, alcohol, chocolate

**S/S:** Heartburn, chest pain, dysphagia and odynophagia, regurgitation, nocturnal aspiration, persistent nonproductive cough, hoarseness (secondary to reflux laryngitis, repetitive throat clearing, hiccups), full feeling in throat, ear pain, loss of dental enamel, night sweats, exacerbation of asthma symptoms

**Red Flags:** N/V, weight loss, bloody stools, true chest pain, dysphagia, anemia, age > 50

**Dx:**
- Endoscopy—if empiric treatment fails or danger signs present
- Barium swallow—1st-line test if obstructive symptoms or danger signs present
- Esophagoscopy—mucosal biopsy
- Manometry—assesses motility and LES function
- Acid reflux test—Ph monitoring of lower esophagus (24-hr test)

**Tx:**
- Lifestyle changes—sleep with head up, lose weight, no food within 3 hr of bedtime; decrease or eliminate ETOH, caffeine, chocolate, fat, mint, no smoking; eliminate medications that ↓ LES tone (calcium channel blockers)
- Medications—antacids, H$_2$ blockers or PPIs, prokinetics (metoclopramide)
- Severe GERD—PPIs indefinitely, surgery (laparoscopic or open fundoplication)

**Complications:** Esophageal ulcers, stricture, bleeding, Barrett's esophagus

## 3.17 HEMOCHROMATOSIS

**Etiology:** Chronic iron overload; patients slowly accumulate iron from infancy but do not exhibit signs for several decades

**S/S:**
- Chronic hepatitis, hepatomegaly, possible cirrhosis (hepatic iron overload)
- Diabetes (pancreatic iron overload)
- CHF, arrhythmias, cardiomyopathy (cardiac iron overload)
- Bronzed skin (iron deposition in skin)
- Adrenal insufficiency, hypogonadism (iron deposits in pituitary)
- Arthritis (iron deposition in joints)

**Dx:** Labs: ↑ serum iron (> 300 mg/dL); ↑ transferrin saturation (> 50%); ↑ serum ferritin and RBC ferritin; ↑ urinary iron excretion; liver biopsy is diagnostic

**Tx:** Weekly phlebotomy until serum iron is normal; iron chelator if patient does not tolerate phlebotomy; treat associated diseases; liver transplant if cirrhosis occurs

**Complications:** Cirrhosis, CHF, hepatocellular carcinoma, arrhythmias, sudden cardiac death

## 3.18 HEPATITIS, ACUTE

**Definition:** Inflammation of the liver, may result in areas of necrosis

**Etiology:** Hepatitis viruses, alcohol, drug-induced, autoimmune disease, EBV, CMV, yellow fever, herpes, rubella, adenovirus, TB, sarcoidosis, IBD, hemochromatosis, Wilson's disease

**S/S:**
- Jaundice, dark urine, pale stools, hepatomegaly, fatigue, malaise, lethargy, RUQ pain, N/V, fever, headache
- Liver failure—edema, hypoalbuminemia, hepatic encephalopathy, hyperestrogenemia, GI bleed

**Dx:** Labs: ↑ AST/ALT and bilirubin; normal to slightly ↑ alkaline phosphatase; ↑ PT/PTT, coagulopathies; hypoalbuminemia; hyperammonemia; viral markers, autoantibody measurements; biopsy may be diagnostic

**Tx:** Removal of offending substance(s); liver transplant for end-stage liver failure; treat acute complications as needed

**Complications:** Multiorgan failure, hepatorenal syndrome, hepatopulmonary syndrome, hepatic encephalopathy, chronic hepatitis, cirrhosis, hepatocellular carcinoma, varices, sepsis

## 3.19 HEPATITIS, CHRONIC

**Definition:** Chronic inflammatory reaction of the liver (greater than 6 months) demonstrated by persistently abnormal LFTs

**Etiology:** Sequela of infection resulting from any cause of acute hepatitis; 2 types:

1. Persistent—benign disorder follows typical acute hepatitis, vague or no symptoms, ALT/AST ↑ but all other LFTs are normal, no physical findings
2. Active (aggressive)—serious disorder, often results in liver failure or cirrhosis; idiopathic origin

**S/S:** One-third of cases follow acute hepatitis, nonspecific malaise, anorexia, fatigue, +/− jaundice, splenomegaly, spider nevi, fluid retention, acne, amenorrhea, arthralgias, ulcerative colitis, pulmonary fibrosis, nephritis, hemolytic anemia

**Dx:** Liver biopsy (essential for definitive diagnosis): periportal necrosis with lymphocytic and plasma cell infiltrates, +/− frank cirrhosis

**Tx:** Avoid causative drugs; manage complications as needed; corticosteroids, +/− azathioprine (for autoimmune types, not as useful for viral cases)

**Complications:** Hepatocellular failure, cirrhosis

## 3.20A HEPATITIS, SPECIFIC TYPES

**Types:**
- Hepatitis A
- Hepatitis B
- Hepatitis C
- Hepatitis D
- Hepatitis E
- Hepatitis AI

**Etiology:**
- A—single-stranded DNA picornavirus; fecal-to-oral transmission; incubation: approx 30 days
- B—enveloped, spherical DNA multiplies via reverse transcription; blood/body fluid; 60–90 days
- C—single-stranded DNA Flavivirus; blood/body fluids; 15–120 days
- D—spherical particle enveloped by HBsAg; can infect only those with HBV; 30–50 days
- E—small, spherical RNA Calicivirus; fecal-to-oral transmission and waterborne; approx 40 days

- AI—viruses, drugs, other chemicals in genetically predisposed patients; loss of tolerance against one's own liver, probably a loss of cell-mediated immunity

**S/S:**
- A—jaundice 2–4 months, N/V, anorexia, ABD pain, diarrhea, arthralgias
- B—chronic viral hepatitis > 6 months histological evidence of inflammation and necrosis
- C—long period without symptoms (+/− 20 yr), then cirrhosis develops
- D—asymptomatic in chronic carriers
- E—same as in other types of viral hepatitis
- AI—abrupt-onset acute hepatitis 50% of the time, the rest with insidious onset; jaundice, anorexia, fatigue, amenorrhea, arthritis, vasculitis, glomerulonephritis, colitis, pericarditis

*(continued)*

## 3.20B HEPATITIS, SPECIFIC TYPES, Continued

**Dx:**
- A—anti-HAV IgM: acute infection; anti-HAV IgG: past exposure (confers immunity)
- B—acute infection: HbsAg +, HBV DNA +, HbeAg (indicates ↑ replication); chronic carrier: HbsAg +, HbeAg −, HBV; chronic disease: HbsAg +, HbeAg +, HBV DNA +
- C—anti-HCV: past exposure; ↑ AST/ALT (2–3 times normal)
- D—anti-HDV IgM or IsG; check for serum markers for HBV
- E—anti-HEV antibodies or HEV RNA
- AI—↑ AST/ALT (usually < 1000); hypergammaglobulinemia (> 2.5 g/dL); cytopenia; PT, bilirubin, and alkaline phosphatase normal early, ↑ late; autoantibodies are often present

**Tx:**
- A—bed rest and symptomatic relief for nausea
- B—interferon α-2b daily for 4 months **OR** lamivudine orally for 1 year; liver transplant for end-stage disease
- C—ribavirin and interferon, avoid alcohol and acetaminophen, correct coagulopathies, maintain hydration and dietary intake
- D—interferon-α for at least 1 year
- E—usually self-limited; prevention is key
- AI—glucocorticoids are mainstay; prednisone 50 mg daily to start, then taper to 10–20 mg daily

**Complications:**
- A—aplastic anemia, fulminant hepatitis
- B—hepatocellular carcinoma, cirrhosis
- C—chronic infection, cirrhosis, hepatocellular carcinoma
- D—chronic hepatitis
- E—pregnant women in 2nd to 3rd trimester have poorest outcomes with approximately 25% mortality, ↑ risk of abortion, stillbirth, neonatal death
- AI—cirrhosis, hepatic failure, encephalopathy, coma, infection, hepatocellular carcinoma

## 3.21 HEPATOCELLULAR CARCINOMA

**Etiology:** Hepatitis B, C, and D; alcoholic liver disease; hemochromatosis; Wilson's disease; *Aspergillus* toxin

**S/S:** Classic presentation—RUQ/epigastric pain, abdominal swelling/ascites, weight loss in a patient with existing cirrhosis, fever, malaise, enlarged hard liver with irregular surface, vascular bruit

**Dx:**
- ↑ alkaline phosphatase; ↑ AFP
- US, CT, or MRI
- Angiography
- Liver biopsy is diagnostic

**Tx:** Surgical resection, removal of liver, and/or liver transplant

**Complications:** Liver failure, death

## 3.22  HIATAL HERNIA

**Types:**
- Sliding (S)
- Paraesophageal (P)

**Etiology:**
- Characterized by widening of the esophageal hiatus of the diaphragm
- S—(95%) an upward dislocation of the gastroesophageal junction; most likely due to age-related stretching of the esophageal hiatus
- P—"rolling" of the gastric fundus upward along a normally positioned cardia; most likely due to congenital hiatal defect

**S/S:**
- S—heartburn, regurgitation, dysphagia
- P—dysphagia, postprandial fullness, heartburn, regurgitation, hematemesis, dyspnea, aspiration and recurrent pneumonia

**Dx:** Upright x-ray—air-fluid level behind cardiac shadow (usually due to P), UGI—near 100% sensitive for P, not as sensitive for S, esophagoscopy—good for either type

**Tx:**
- S—treat as GERD
- P—surgery is only effective treatment

**Complications:** Ulceration of the herniated fundus, aspiration pneumonia

## 3.23  HYPERTROPHIC PYLORIC STENOSIS

**Etiology:** Gastric outlet obstruction, occurs in first 2 months of life, peak incidence 2–4 weeks with M:F ratio 4:1

**S/S:**
- Projectile nonbilious vomiting, dehydration, poor weight gain, hypokalemic, hypochloremic metabolic alkalosis
- Classic findings—olive-sized, muscular, mobile, nontender epigastric mass, +/− peristaltic waves

**Dx:** Labs—electrolytes; US, hypertrophic pylorus

**Tx:** NG tube, correct dehydration, electrolytes abnormalities, and alkalosis; pyloromyotomy is curative

**Complications:** Failure to thrive, death

## 3.24 INTUSSUSCEPTION

**Etiology:** Telescoping of one part of the intestine into another; among the most common causes of bowel obstruction in infancy

**S/S:** Violent episodes of irritability, colicky pain, and emesis interspersed with normal periods, rectal bleeding, tubular mass on palpation

**Dx:**
- ABD x-ray—air fluid levels
- BE or air enema—"coiled-spring" appearance to bowel

**Tx:**
- Fluid resuscitation
- BE or air enema will reduce 75% of cases if done within the first 48 hr
- Laparotomy with direct reduction if unreduced by BE or air enema or if peritoneal signs are present

**Complications:** Recurrence

## 3.25 IRRITABLE BOWEL SYNDROME

**Etiology:** Motility disorder involving the small intestine and large bowel associated with variable degrees of abdominal pain, constipation or diarrhea, dyspeptic symptoms; often precipitated by ↑ stress and anxiety

**S/S:** Diffuse abdominal tenderness, flatulence, nausea, anorexia, HA, fatigue, lassitude, erratic frequency of bowel action and variation in stool consistency

**Dx:**
- Stool exam—occult blood, O&P, culture, leukocytes
- Proctosigmoidoscopy—evaluate for polyps or neoplasms
- Labs—CBC, ESR, chem panel (including amylase), UA
- ABD US, BE, UGI with SBFT for selected patients

**Tx:**
- Supportive and palliative—must first assure no organic cause for symptoms exist
- Dietary changes—may or may not be helpful, each patient should determine if specific foods trigger attacks
- Bulking agents, antispasmodics, antidiarrheals, antidepressants

**Complications:** Psychosocial issues (job, family)

## 3.26 JAUNDICE OF INFANCY

**Types:** (Most common benign causes of jaundice in infancy)
- Physiologic (P)
- Breast milk–induced (B)

**Etiology:**
- P—a transient, unconjugated hyperbilirubinemia during the 1st week of life; due to increased RBC volume, decreased RBC survival time, and increased enterohepatic circulation
- B—unknown factor in breast milk

**S/S:**
- P—begins after 24 hr of life, peaks at day 3 with bilirubin level 12–15 mg/dL and returns to normal by end of first week
- B—peak bilirubin level is higher than with physiologic, otherwise appears very similar

**Dx:** CBC with peripheral smear, Coombs' test, conjugated and unconjugated levels

**Tx:**
- P—phototherapy (controversial when to start); severe cases, exchange therapy
- B—stop breast-feeding

**Complications:** Kernicterus, sublethal bilirubin encephalopathy

## 3.27 LIVER ABSCESS

**Etiology:** *Entamoeba histolytica* or bacteria most common causes; liver infection usually secondary to bacteremia, ascending cholangitis, or penetrating trauma

**S/S:** Intense, constant RUQ pain, +/− radiation to right shoulder; ↑ pain with cough, deep breathing or lying on right side; fever, chills, night sweats

**Dx:**
- Labs—leukocytosis > 15,000
- ↑ alkaline phosphatase and transaminases
- Antiamebic serum antibody present in > 90% of patients
- Mild anemia, ↑ bilirubin
- RUQ US is test of choice

**Tx:** Metronidazole for 2 weeks for *E. histolytica;* broad-spectrum antibiotics for all bacterial infections; percutaneous drainage of abscess; surgical drainage for rupture abscess

**Complications:** Rupture, subphrenic abscess

## 3.28 MALABSORPTION SYNDROMES

**Types:**
- Abnormal digestion (AD)
- Impaired absorption (IA)

**Etiology:**
- AD—malabsorption of 1 or many nutrients due to insufficient gastric mixing (gastrectomy); ↓ enzymes (CF, pancreatitis, liver failure, lactase or IF deficiency); ↓ acidity (Z-E syndrome, subtotal gastrectomy)
- IA—due to damaged absorptive surface (infection, sprue, Whipple's disease, alcohol, drugs, amyloidosis, Crohn's disease, ischemic colitis); ↓ absorptive surface (resection, infarcted bowel, volvulus)

**S/S:** Osmotic diarrhea and steatorrhea; bulky, greasy stools; bloating, distention, flatus; weight loss, anorexia; glossitis, carpopedal spasm; vitamin and mineral deficiencies; amenorrhea (fat ↓); osteopenia (ca/vit D ↓); tetany (ca ↓); coagulation disorders (vit K ↓); neuropathy (vit $B_{12}$ ↓); edema and ascites (protein ↓)

**Dx:**
- 72-hr fecal fat analysis
- Xylose absorption test (intestinal absorptive capacity)
- Intestinal biopsy and cultures (infection, CA, patency of absorptive surface)
- Small bowel follow-through (sprue, Whipple's disease, fistulas, stasis, blind loop, diverticulosis, Crohn's disease)
- Pancreatic function test
- $H_2$ breath test (lactose intolerance)
- Schilling test (vit $B_{12}$)
- Obtain levels for iron, folate, gastrin (Z-E syndrome)
- Cortisol (Addison's disease)
- Sweat chloride (CF)

**Tx:** Treat underlying disorder

**Complications:** Malnutrition, failure to thrive, death

## 3.29 MALLORY-WEISS SYNDROME

**Etiology:** Longitudinal, partial-thickness tear at the level of the gastroesophageal junction, may extend into the stomach. Follows a prolonged period of severe vomiting and retching

**S/S:** Hematemesis following vomiting, straining, or coughing; bright red blood, generally mild and self-limited; +/− chest pain

**Dx:** Clinical diagnosis, endoscopy to confirm and treat

**Tx:**
- Supportive—volume replacement, gastric lavage, vasoconstrictive medication
- During endoscopy—direct electrocautery or epinephrine injection
- Exploratory laparotomy if bleeding persists or rupture suspected

**Complications:** Infection, ulcer formation, recurrence (if treated nonoperatively), rupture

## 3.30 OBESITY

**Etiology:** An excess of adipose tissue, measured by BMI

BMI = measured body weight in kg divided by height in meters squared; normal = 20–25 kg/m$^2$; less than 1% of obese patients have an identifiable secondary cause (hypothyroidism or Cushing's syndrome)

**S/S:**
- Mild obesity—BMI 27.5–30 kg/m$^2$
- Moderate obesity—BMI 30–40 kg/m$^2$
- Morbid obesity—BMI > 40 kg/m$^2$

**Dx:**
- Detailed H&P to include age at onset, recent weight changes, family history of obesity, occupational history, eating and exercise behavior, cigarette and alcohol use, and psychosocial issues
- Labs—endocrinologic panel including dexamethasone suppression test and TSH

**Tx:** Multidisciplinary approach with hypocaloric diets, behavior modification, aerobic exercise and social support; medications may have short-term advantages; surgical therapy should be considered last resort

**Complications:** Diabetes mellitus, hypertension, cardiovascular disease, pulmonary disease, death

## 3.31 PANCREATIC CARCINOMA

**Etiology:** Smoking, mutations in K-*ras;* > 95% are adenocarcinoma

**S/S:** Insidious onset of weight loss, fatigue, anorexia, gnawing abdominal and back pain; epigastric pain radiating to back, may improve with leaning forward; painless jaundice; dark urine, pale stools; COURVOISIER'S SIGN, diabetes mellitus, migratory thrombophlebitis

**Dx:**
- Labs—↑ CEA and CA 19-9; ↑ alkaline phosphatase and bilirubin (if liver mets or bile duct obstruction)
- CT of abdomen
- Percutaneous or open biopsy for tissue diagnosis

**Tx:**
- Resection—the only effective treatment
- Chemotherapy may increase survival
- Radiation therapy for palliative treatment only
- Pain control, pancreatic enzyme replacement for quality of life

**Complications:** Widespread mets; 90% of cases will have metastasized by the time of diagnosis

## 3.32 PANCREATITIS, CHRONIC

**Etiology:** Alcohol abuse is most common; other causes include hyperparathyroidism, cystic fibrosis, severe protein-calorie malnutrition, obstruction of pancreatic duct, idiopathic

**S/S:** Chronic epigastric pain radiating to back; steatorrhea, signs of malnutrition, jaundice, glucose intolerance

**Dx:**
- Classic triad—pancreatic calcification, steatorrhea, diabetes
- Labs—amylase and lipase normal, vitamin $B_{12}$ deficiency
- ERCP or MRCP—"gold standard"
- US or CT—not as good
- ABD x-ray—calcification of the pancreas in 1/3 of cases

**Tx:**
- Avoid alcohol and fatty foods
- Replace enzymes and vitamins $B_{12}$, A, D, E, and K
- Antacids, $H_2$ blockers, pain control
- Local resection or ductal dilation
- Insulin or hypoglycemic agent if diabetes is present

**Complications:** Pancreatic cancer

## 3.33 PEPTIC ULCER DISEASE

**Etiology:**
- Duodenal ulcers—*H. pylori* infection (75%), Z-E syndrome (3–5%)
- Gastric—steroids and NSAIDs
- Gastrinoma (causes ↑ acid production), +/− Crohn's disease, smoking, personality and stress

**S/S:**
- Gnawing/burning epigastric or RUQ pain, +/− hematemesis/melena
- Pain response to eating—G, ↑ pain with meal; D, initial ↓ pain but 2–3 hr after meal, pain ↑
- Perforated—severe pain with rebound tenderness to palpation and guarding

**Dx:**
- Endoscopy with biopsy
- UGI series—less sensitive and specific, misses angiodysplasia
- Suspected perforation—upright ABD x-ray shows free air under diaphragm

**Tx:**
- Eradicate *H. pylori*—triple therapy; antacids, $H_2$ blockers, PPIs; sucralfate (mucosal protectant agent)
- Eliminate exacerbating factors (smoking, ETOH, NSAIDs)
- Surgery (indicated for intractable bleeding, gastric outlet obstruction, perforation, Z-E syndrome)

**Complications:** Malignant transformation, massive blood loss, peritonitis, infection, death

## 3.34 SCLEROSING CHOLANGITIS, PRIMARY

**Etiology:** A premalignant condition of the biliary tree characterized by inflammation, fibrosis, stenosing of the bile ducts for unknown reasons; secondary sclerosing cholangitis causes bile duct injury or bile duct ischemia

**S/S:** RUQ pain, jaundice, pruritus, fatigue, nausea, +/− S/S of <u>ULCERATIVE COLITIS</u> or <u>CROHN'S DISEASE</u>

**Dx:**
- ERCP is "gold standard"
- Labs—↑ alkaline phosphatase for over 6 months
- Hypergammaglobulinemia; ↑ ANA/AMA/ASMA possible

**Tx:**
- No medical treatment is effective
- Stent placement and biliary drainage relieve or ↓ symptoms but do not improve mortality
- Antibiotics to treat superimposed bacterial infection
- Liver transplant is curative

**Complications:** Recurrence (20% will recur after transplant), liver failure, acute cholangitis

## 3.35 SCURVY

**Etiology:** Vitamin C deficiency, in USA usually due to dietary inadequacy

**S/S:** Malaise, weakness, perifollicular hemorrhages, perifollicular hyperkeratotic papules, petechiae and purpura, splinter hemorrhages, bleeding gums, joint hemorrhages, subperiosteal hemorrhages, anemia, edema, oliguria, neuropathy, intracerebral hemorrhage

**Dx:** Clinical diagnosis, confirmed with decreased plasma levels of vitamin C

**Tx:** 100–300 mg of ascorbic acid per day

**Complications:** Vitamin C toxicity (rare), gastric irritation, flatulence, diarrhea

## 3.36 TOXIC MEGACOLON

**Etiology:** Results from extensive damage to the colonic mucosa with areas of mucosal denudation and inflammation of the submucosal layers

**S/S:** Evidence of systemic toxicity, fever, leukocytosis, tachycardia, ABD distention

**Dx:** ABD x-ray shows dilated colon

**Tx:**
- Decompress the bowel and pass an intestinal tube to prevent swallowed air from further distending the colon
- Replace lost fluids and electrolytes
- Restore colloid and blood volume
- Hydrocortisone; broad-spectrum antibiotics
- Surgical—colectomy if colon does not decompress with medical treatment

**Complications:** Sepsis, death

## 3.37 ULCERATIVE COLITIS

**Etiology:** Idiopathic, chronic, relapsing inflammatory disorder of rectum and colon

**S/S:** Intermittent bouts of bloody, mucous diarrhea with periods of constipation; lower ABD pain and cramps relieved by defecation; +/− fever, weight loss, tenesmus, and constipation with proctitis; failure to thrive in children

**Dx:**
- Colonoscopy with biopsy is diagnostic
- BE—ulceration, pseudopolyps, "lead pipe" appearance of colon in end-stage cases
- UGI with SBFT
- Proctoscopy, stool culture

**Tx:**
- Daily—sulfasalazine, mesalamine, hydrocortisone enema, antidiarrheals and bulking agents
- Flare-ups—bowel rest (NPO, NGT), IV fluids, steroids, metronidazole
- Colectomy—curative
- Indications for surgery—dysplasia/CA, perforation, toxic colitis, hemorrhage, intractable disease, inability to wean off steroids

**Complications:** Toxic megacolon, strictures, obstruction, perforation, hypokalemia, hemorrhage, shock, colon CA

CHAPTER 4

# Musculoskeletal System

## 4.1 ADHESIVE CAPSULITIS

**Etiology:**
- Uncertain; some type of inflammatory process about the shoulder → progressive limitation in ROM
- 3 phases—1st, inflammation → scar formation within the capsule; 2nd, shoulder has undergone fibrous arthrodesis → stiffness; 3rd, stiffness resolves → progressive improvement in ROM

**S/S:** Night pain, ↓ PROM and AROM, ↑ pain at extremes of ROM with firm endpoint

**Dx:** Clinical diagnosis, x-rays = +/− disuse osteopenia

**Tx:**
- PT for ROM exercises and stretching
- MUA if no improvement after 3+ months
- Surgical capsular release is controversial, may be arthroscopic or open

**Complications:** Humeral fracture, glenohumeral dislocation, rotator cuff tears, radial nerve injury (all usually 2° to overly aggressive MUA)

## 4.2 ANKLE FRACTURE

**Etiology:** May involve tibia (medial or posterior malleoli), fibula (lateral malleolus), talus (anterior lip)

**S/S:**
- Inversion or eversion injury, immediate pain, swelling and inability to bear weight, +/− deformity
- P/E—TTP over ankle, +/− abnormal motion/crepitus about bony structures, must assess entire length of fibula to evaluate for MAISONNEUVE'S FRACTURE; many classification systems for ankle fractures

**Dx:** X-ray is diagnostic for most, *must* have at least 3 views (AP, lat, mortise)

**Tx:** Most medial malleolus fractures require ORIF; lateral malleolus fractures require ORIF if syndesmosis is unstable; if stable and fracture is non- or minimally displaced, may treat in cast NWB × 6 weeks; syndesmosis disruption (Maisonneuve injury) requires syndesmotic screws

**Complications:** Nonunion, malunion, soft tissue slough, infection, RSD, posttraumatic osteoarthritis

## 4.3  ANKLE SPRAIN

**Etiology:**
- Sprain is injury to ligament at a joint
- Strain is injury to tendon or muscle (treatment and workup the same)

**S/S:** History of "rolling over" ankle, graded I–III
- Grade I—stretching of ligament without tear, usually single ligament; P/E: minimal swelling, point tenderness without instability or loss of function
- Grade II—partial tear of ligament, usually ATFL +/− CFL involved; P/E: significant swelling, TTP, and ↓ ROM, +/− positive anterior drawer or TALAR TILT TEST
- Grade III—complete disruption of ligament, involves 2 or more ligaments; P/E: extensive swelling, ecchymosis, TTP about ankle, inability to bear weight, +/− instability (hard to demonstrate due to guarding against exam 2° to pain), muscle spasm

**Dx:** X-ray: according to OTTAWA ANKLE RULES, +/− stress radiographs if instability is suspected

**Tx:** RICE protocol (rest, ice, compression, elevation), restrict weight bearing to patient's tolerance, NSAIDs, PT once initial symptoms ↓ (ROM, gait, strengthening, proprioception training)

**Complications:** Chronic lateral ankle instability

## 4.4  ANKYLOSING SPONDYLITIS

**Etiology:** An inflammatory polyarthropathy characterized by sacroiliitis and the presence of HLA-B27

**S/S:** Low back pain worse in the morning, improves as day goes on; ↓ ROM to spine; sacroiliitis (tender SI joints)

**Dx:**
- X-ray—bilateral sacroiliitis, "bamboo spine" (late finding)
- Labs—↑ ESR; + HLA-B27

**Tx:**
- NSAIDs for pain control, intra-articular corticosteroid injections
- Azulfidine, methotrexate
- Physical therapy with emphasis on extension exercises

**Complications:** Severe hip arthritis, spinal fractures, secondary amyloidosis, apical pulmonary fibrosis, complications secondary to NSAIDs

## 4.5 ANTERIOR CRUCIATE LIGAMENT (ACL) INJURY

**Etiology:** May be related to anatomic variations in the intercondylar notch of the distal femur, ligament size, muscular strength, neuromuscular control, and hormonal influences

**S/S:**
- History of deceleration injury +/− valgus rotation and/or hyperextension; feeling a pop or snap, inability to bear weight, swelling over short period of time (hours, not days)
- P/E—Moderate to severe effusion, + LACHMAN'S TEST, + anterior drawer, + PIVOT SHIFT TEST

**Dx:** X-rays: usually normal, +/− SEGOND FRACTURE (pathognomonic); MRI is diagnostic

**Tx:**
- Individualized to the patient based on extent of injury, functional goals, and expectations; first step is to regain full ROM, quadriceps strength, and complete resolution of effusion
- Nonoperative: PT, bracing, activity modification
- Operative: reconstruction, requires extensive rehab after surgery → ROM → strengthening → sports-specific training (takes 3–6 months)

**Complications:** Persistent instability, stiffness or weakness, graft failure with rerupture

## 4.6 AVASCULAR NECROSIS

**Etiology:**
- Infarction and necrosis of bone marrow, trabecular bone, and subchondral bone due to compromised blood supply
- Common causes—trauma, corticosteroid use, alcohol abuse, sickle cell anemia, radiation therapy, Gaucher's disease, decompression injury, pancreatitis, hyperlipidemia, thrombosis

**S/S:** Severe pain, ↓ with rest; limited and painful ROM; noninflammatory joint effusion

**Dx:** X-rays: irregular contour of joint articulation (very late in course of disease when changes seen on x-rays); MRI or bone scan better early tests

**Tx:**
- Early stages—limited weight bearing and analgesics
- Surgical options—core decompression; osteotomy and bone grafting; total joint replacement; joint fusion

**Complications:** Arthritis, limited mobility

## 4.7  BLOUNT'S DISEASE

**Etiology:** Tibia vara—poorly understood loss of medial tibial physeal growth → progressive bowing of the leg, early walking in heavy children with physiologic bowing may contribute; ↑ incidence in black and Hispanic children; adolescent type may be associated with trauma

**S/S:** Nonpainful bowing of legs, may be unilateral or bilateral, usually presents between 2 and 4 years of age for infantile and juvenile types, may appear in adolescence (posttraumatic)

**Dx:** X-ray: decreased medial tibial physeal growth +/− distortion of the medial articular surface and fusion of the physis

**Tx:**
- Mild cases—no treatment needed
- Severe or progressive cases—surgical correction

**Complications:** Physeal bridging requiring repeated surgical correction of angular deformity, leg-length inequality, delayed union, compartment syndromes, peroneal nerve palsy

## 4.8  CARPAL TUNNEL SYNDROME

**Etiology:**
- Space-occupying lesions—fracture fragments, dislocated carpal bones, ganglion, tumor
- Medical conditions—DM, collagen diseases, amyloidosis, hormonal changes (menopause, pregnancy)
- Repetitive motion (occupational or recreational)

**S/S:** Pain and paresthesias to the median nerve distribution, nocturnal paresthesias, difficulty holding or dropping objects, + Tinel and Phalen's tests

**Dx:** Clinical diagnosis confirmed by EMG (may be false negative up to 20% of time)

**Tx:**
- Conservative—rest, wrist splint, NSAIDs, +/− steroid injection
- Surgical—open or endoscopic carpal tunnel release

**Complications:** Stenosing tenosynovitis (trigger finger or thumb), permanent nerve damage (from long-standing CTS or surgical complication), recurrence

## 4.9 CLUBFOOT DEFORMITY

**Etiology:** Congenital talipes equinovarus = severe fixed deformity of the foot characterized by ankle plantarflexion (equinus), inversion and axial IR of the subtalar (talocalcaneal) joint (varus), and medial subluxation of the talonavicular and calcaneocuboid joints (adductus)

**S/S:** Rigid deformity as described above +/− severe cavus with medial and plantar midfoot crease

**Dx:** X-ray rarely of value initially, becomes more important if surgical intervention is planned or if the child does not present until walking

**Tx:**
- Conservative—begins at birth; parents are taught passive manipulation and positioning to correct deformity; serial manipulation and casting started by 1 week and continues each wk for 1 month then every 1–2 weeks for 2–3 months
- Surgical—persistent deformity after serial casting once age 3–6 months

**Complications:** Recurrent deformity, incompletely corrected deformity at surgery, overcorrection of deformity

## 4.10 COLLES' FRACTURE

**Etiology:**
- Fall onto outstretched hand
- Classic fracture occurs in skeletally mature person at the metaphyseal-diaphyseal junction of the distal radius; it is extra-articular, dorsally displaced/angulated

**S/S:** Pain/swelling, deformity ("dinner fork"), ↓ ROM to digits and wrist 2° to pain

**Dx:** X-rays reveal fracture as described above

**Tx:** Closed reduction and casting in clinic or ED; if it fails (closed reduction or adequate reduction not obtained), proceed with closed reduction and pinning under anesthesia; ORIF rarely required

**Complications:** Median nerve dysfunction; compartment syndrome; stiffness of shoulder, elbow, wrist, or fingers; malunion or nonunion (rare); delayed rupture of extensor pollicis longus; CTS; RSD; distal radioulnar joint dysfunction

## 4.11 CUBITAL TUNNEL SYNDROME

**Etiology:** Compression of the ulnar nerve along the medial elbow between the ulnar and humeral origins of the flexor carpi ulnaris or at the proximal border of the cubital tunnel due to stretching with elbow flexion

**S/S:**
- Paresthesia and numbness to the small and ulnar half of the ring finger, ↑ with full flexion of the elbow
- +/− night pain that wakes patient
- + Tinel sign
- Motor weakness to first dorsal interosseous muscle and flexor digitorum profundus to the small finger
- + FROMENT'S SIGN
- + elbow flexion test (paresthesia within 60 sec of elbow flexion)

**Dx:** Clinical diagnosis, confirmed by EMG

**Tx:**
- Conservative—elbow pad, elbow splint at night to prevent flexion > 45°, NSAIDs, corticosteroid injections
- Surgical—decompression +/− anterior transposition of the nerve, +/− medial epicondylectomy

**Complications:** Recurrence, residual motor weakness after decompression (usually due to severity of condition before surgery)

## 4.12 DE QUERVAIN'S TENOSYNOVITIS

**Etiology:** Inflammation of the tendons of the first dorsal compartment (APL & EPB)

**S/S:** Pain over the radial aspect of the wrist, + FINKELSTEIN'S TEST

**Dx:** Clinical diagnosis

**Tx:**
- Rest, NSAIDs, thumb spica splinting
- Cortisone injection for refractory cases
- Surgical decompression of the entire first compartment as last resort for chronic cases

**Complications:** Chronic pain

## 4.13 DYSPLASIA OF THE HIP, DEVELOPMENTAL

**Etiology:** Multifactorial—genetic, ethnic, mechanical, hormonal factors involved

**S/S:**
- Birth to 2 months of age—+ ORTOLANI and/or BARLOW TESTS
- 2 months to walking age—↓ abduction of affected hip, asymmetrical skin folds, + GALEAZZI'S SIGN
- Walking age and beyond—TRENDELENBURG GAIT

**Dx:**
- US—more reliable from birth to 4 months
- X-ray—after age 4 months, normal bony anatomy better developed, making plain films more reliable

**Tx: Age-related:**
- Birth–6 months—Pavlik harness; if dislocation persists after 4 consecutive weeks, proceed to CR and spica casting
- 6–18 mo—traction for 2–3 weeks → closed reduction and spica casting, +/– adductor tenotomy
- 18 mo–3 yrs—open reduction +/– varus derotational osteotomy of the proximal femur and spica casting
- 3–8 yrs—open reduction, femoral shortening, varus derotational osteotomy + pelvic osteotomy
- Over 8 yrs—controversial, some recommend nonoperative care, others favor triple osteotomies

**Complications:** AVN of the femoral head, DJD of hip

## 4.14 EPICONDYLITIS, LATERAL

**Etiology:** Overuse involving continuous flexion/extension of the elbow in combination with pronation/supination of the forearm → microtrauma to the extensor carpi radialis brevis tendon

**S/S:**
- Pain over the lateral epicondyle +/– radiation to forearm; +/– wrist and hand weakness with grasping; pain with "power grip" or grasping with wrist in extension
- P/E—point tenderness over lateral epicondyle (over insertion of the ECRB), pain ↑ with resisted wrist and long finger extension with the elbow in full extension and forearm in full pronation, + "COFFEE CUP" TEST

**Dx:** Clinical diagnosis

**Tx:** NSAIDs, avoid aggravating activity, ice (initial stages), +/– corticosteroid injection, counterforce bracing; surgery for severe symptoms that do not respond to conservative care

**Complications:** Chronic pain

## 4.15 EPICONDYLITIS, MEDIAL

**Etiology:** Inflammation of the flexor pronator mass, specifically the pronator teres and flexor carpi radialis

**S/S:**
- Usually insidious onset of pain, pain radiates along medial elbow, +/− ache over flexor/pronator mass, weak grip strength, +/− ulnar nerve irritation
- P/E—tenderness over flexor pronator origin (pronator teres and FCR), pain ↑ with resisted wrist flexion and forearm pronation, +/− Tinel's sign over cubital tunnel

**Dx:** Clinical diagnosis

**Tx:** NSAIDs, rest, local modalities (US, heat), +/− corticosteroid injections; surgical release for refractory cases

**Complications:** Persistent pain or weakness

## 4.16 FIBROMYALGIA

**Definition:** A group of common nonarticular rheumatic disorders, may be of primary or secondary type

**Etiology:** Pain in the fibrous connective tissue, may be induced or intensified by physical or mental stress, poor sleep, trauma, exposure to dampness or cold, or a systemic disorder

**S/S:** Pain, tenderness, stiffness of muscles and areas of tendon insertions (trigger points), pain ↑ by overuse, straining, poor sleep, anxiety, fatigue, IBS

**Dx:**
- Clinical exam and exclusion of other systemic diseases
- Labs: ANA, RA, ESR, CRP

**Tx:**
- Supportive measures—reassurance, explanation of benign nature of disease
- Stretching exercises, improved sleep, heat, gentle massage, low-dose tricyclic antidepressant at bedtime, ASA or other NSAID, trigger-point injections

**Complications:** None

## 4.17 GANGLION CYST

**Etiology:** Varies by site, can originate from tendon, bone, or any joint on the hand/wrist or foot/ankle; often associated with inflammatory or degenerative arthritis

**S/S:** Mass, +/− pain, discomfort, weakness, restricted motion, disfigurement; mass is usually firm and immobile, may fluctuate in size

**Dx:** Clinical diagnosis

**Tx:** Needle aspiration may decrease size, but recurrence is common; surgical excision is associated with recurrence rate of less than 10% if entire capsule is removed

**Complications:** CTS, recurrence

## 4.18 GOUT

**Etiology:** A syndrome—hyperuricemia → monosodium urate crystal formation → inflammation → tissue injury → tophi and arthritis

**S/S:** Acute gouty arthritis: repeated attacks of severe joint pain, swelling, erythema; PODAGRA; +/− fever

**Dx:**
- Aspiration of synovial fluid or tophi is diagnostic
- X-rays: MARTEL'S SIGN

**Tx:** For acute attacks:
- Indomethacin and other NSAIDs
- Oral colchicines
- Corticosteroids in severe disease
- Avoid hypouricemic treatment (allopurinol)
- Prophylaxis—allopurinol; low-dose colchicines; uricosuric drugs (probenecid, sulfinpyrazone)

**Complications:** Chronic destructive arthropathy

## 4.19  HAND INFECTIONS: FELON

**Etiology:**
- Infection of the pulp space of the digit
- Usually results from a puncture wound of the fat pad on the volar aspect of the distal phalanx
- *Staph. aureus* is most common pathogen

**S/S:** Swelling and extreme pain to tip of finger; pain is localized to volar aspect of digit, ↑ with palpation, +/− fluctuance, erythema

**Dx:** Clinical diagnosis

**Tx:** Incision and drainage, requires packing to keep skin open and allow wound to close by secondary intention, oral antibiotics for 7–10 days

**Complications:** Need for repeat I&D, extension of the infection to the flexor tendon sheath, necrosis with osteomyelitis of the distal phalanx

## 4.20  HAND INFECTIONS: FLEXOR TENOSYNOVITIS

**Etiology:**
- Purulent discharge within the flexor tendon sheath of the hand
- May be due to direct inoculation of the tendon sheath or delayed inoculation from a neighboring pathologic process
- *Staph. aureus* is the most common pathogen

**S/S:** KANAVEL'S SIGNS are the cardinal signs

**Dx:** Clinical diagnosis

**Tx:**
- Surgical I&D with catheter placement within the tendon sheath. Catheter is left in place with continuous irrigation for 72 hr, then removed.
- IV antibiotics for 3 to 5 days +/− oral antibiotics
- Most patients require OT to help with ROM to digit

**Complications:** Extension of infection to other digits, tendon necrosis, fibrous adhesions with loss of motion; amputation

## 4.21 HERNIATED NUCLEUS PULPOSUS

**Etiology:** Three classes:
- Protruded—herniated disk material is covered by some amount of intact posterior annulus and PLL
- Extruded—herniated material is in continuity with the disk space but extends into epidural space 2° to rupture of PLL
- Sequestered—herniated disk material free-floating in the epidural space with no continuity to the disk space

**S/S:**
- Lumbar—severe radiating LE pain following a dermatomal pattern depending on the level involved; antalgic gait, painful leg held flexed and patient reluctant to place foot flat on floor when standing; +/− paravertebral muscle spasm; loss of normal lumbar lordosis; ↓ ROM to spine + straight leg raise
- Cervical—HA, neck pain, radiculopathy, myelopathy

**Dx:**
- X-rays—reveal DJD, spondylolysis, spondylolisthesis
- MRI—diagnostic in most cases
- CT myelogram—indicated for patients unable to undergo MRI
- EMG—better for cervical than lumbar radiculopathy

**Tx:**
- Nonoperative—2–3 days' rest, then progressive mobilization, NSAIDs, home exercise program, epidural steroid injections, tapered-dose oral steroids
- Operative—decompression: discectomy, laminotomy, laminectomy

**Complications:** Nerve root injury (with operative treatment), recurrent disk herniation

## 4.22 LEGG-CALVÉ-PERTHES DISEASE

**Etiology:** Ischemia of the femoral head for unknown reasons, affects those 2–13 Y/O, M>F (4:1)

**S/S:** Limp, +/− thigh or knee pain, limited and painful hip motion with ↓ IR and abduction

**Dx:**
- X-rays—normal initially, progress to characteristic collapse of portions of the femoral head
- Signs of head at risk—calcification lateral to epiphysis; diffuse metaphyseal rarefaction; lateral extrusion of the head; growth disturbance of the physis; rarefaction in lateral part of the epiphysis and subjacent metaphysis

**Tx:** Goal: Prevention of deformity of femoral head, usually achieved by containment of head in acetabulum and active motion
- < 6 years—traction, no weight bearing, NSAIDs
- 6–8 years—containment methods (brace, femoral or pelvic osteotomy)
- > 9 years—femoral or pelvic osteotomy

**Complications:** Residual asymmetry of the femoral head and acetabulum, degenerative OA

## 4.23A  LOW BACK PAIN

**Etiology:** Five types
- Arthritic—OA/DJD, RA, spondyloarthropathies
- Mechanical—spondylolisthesis, muscular, fracture, disk/facet disease
- Postural—osteoporosis/poor posture
- Myofascial—muscle cocontraction (→ lactic acid buildup → crampy pain)
- Idiopathic—malignancy, infection, referred pain, unknown

**S/S:**
- OA/DJD—stiffness and soreness after activity, ↓ with rest; AM pain (upon wakening)
- Spondyloarthropathies—early age of onset; pain with rest, improves with activity; ↓ ROM to spine
- Mechanical—pain with motion, improves with rest; +/– <u>RADICULOPATHY</u>
- Postural—progressive pain with activity, ↑ throughout day, relief with rest
- Myofascial—aching, stiffness, soreness with inactivity, better with activity; pain ↑ throughout day and with stress; pain not relieved by rest; + pain with palpation of soft tissues
- **Red Flags:** Fever; trauma; age > 50 or < 20; drug use; refractory to treatment; history of cancer; incontinence; progressive neurologic deficits; weight loss; night pain; impotence

**Dx:** Clinical diagnosis; imaging studies only if red flags are present:
- X-ray—osteomyelitis, cancer, fractures, ankylosing spondylitis, segmental instability
- CT/MRI—disk herniation, stenosis, cauda equina tumors, epidural masses
- Bone scan—osteomyelitis, metastases
- Diskography—Discogenic back pain; EMG/nerve conduction studies for peripheral nerve injuries

*(continued)*

## 4.23B  LOW BACK PAIN, Continued

**Tx:** If red flag signs are present, must do necessary workup with appropriate referral
- Short-term rest for acute pain—no more than 3 days' total rest before beginning activity
- Pain control—nonnarcotic pain medication for chronic pain, short-term use of narcotics appropriate for acute pain only
- Muscle relaxants—no proven benefit, not indicated for long-term use; may help for relief of spasm only (not pain control) in acute injury
- Epidural corticosteroid injections—for radiculopathy
- Patient education—most important aspect of treatment regardless of etiology
- Physical therapy—for education on home exercise program, biomechanics, and limited use of modalities
- Surgery—an option only if patient's symptoms correlate with any pathology found on imaging studies (herniated disk, severe stenosis, fractures, tumors)

**Complications:** Chronic condition, may worsen with time; neurologic deficits; complications of treatment are most common complication (drug addiction, worse postoperative pain, infections)

## 4.24  MALLET FINGER

**Etiology:** Sudden flexion force on an extended distal joint, causes disruption of the terminal end of the extensor mechanism. May be midsubstance or bony (with avulsion fracture)

**S/S:** DIP joint held in flexed position with no active extension

**Dx:** X-rays: +/− dorsal lip avulsion fracture fragment from the distal phalanx at its base

**Tx:**
- Extension splint for 6 wks
- Surgical repair of the tendon for open injuries or pinning of large fracture fragments
- Fusion for chronic deformity

**Complications:** Chronic mallet deformity

## 4.25  MEDIAL COLLATERAL LIGAMENT INJURIES

**Etiology:** Usually abduction injury with associated torsional component; may be isolated or combined injury; most common associated injuries: ACL, lateral tibial plateau fracture, medial>lateral meniscus

**S/S:**
- History of a valgus stress injury
- P/E: TTP about medial knee, laxity with valgus stress, graded on millimeters of laxity (I = 0–5 mm; II = 5–10 mm; III = 10–15 mm)

**Dx:** X-rays may be normal, PELLEGRINI–STIEDA SIGN; MRI is diagnostic

**Tx:**
- Nonoperative is treatment of choice
- Grades I & II—+/− hinged knee brace, protected weight bearing
- Grade III—long leg hinged knee brace locked at 30° for 2 weeks, then 30°–90° motion for total of 6 weeks

**Complications:** Valgus instability

## 4.26  MENISCAL INJURY

**Etiology:** Rotation with or without axial compression is typical mechanism of injury; also may be due to degenerative injuries or secondary to ACL-deficient knees

**S/S:** Pain, swelling, popping, snapping, locking, effusion, ↓ ROM; P/E: joint-line tenderness, + <u>MCMURRAY'S</u> <u>TEST</u>, + <u>APLEY</u> <u>GRIND</u> <u>TEST</u>

**Dx:** X-ray may be normal; MRI is diagnostic for most

**Tx:**
- Individualized to each patient based on degree of disability and functional goals
- Nonoperative—therapeutic modalities for ↓ swelling, ↑ ROM, balanced strengthening
- Operative—arthroscopic débridement; on rare occasions repair may be possible (peripheral tears in young patients only)

**Complications:** Retear, degenerative joint disease, persistent pain, Baker's cyst

## 4.27  METASTATIC DISEASE TO BONE

**Etiology:** Most common primary tumors that metastasize to bone are breast, lung, thyroid, prostate, kidney ("BLT with pickles and ketchup"); most common location is spine, pelvis, femur, rib, proximal humerus, skull

**S/S:**
- Pain, insidious onset, gradually ↑ in severity over weeks to months
- Long bone mets may produce mechanical symptoms and pain ↑ with use and ↓ with rest
- Constitutional symptoms—anorexia, dehydration, anemia, hypercalcemia

**Dx:**
- Plain x-ray will show most once they are fairly advanced, will not pick up early mets
- Total body bone scan—initial test of choice for screening, will show early mets
- CT scan—determines extent of intra- and extramedullary involvement
- MRI—better at demonstrating extent of marrow or soft tissue involvement

**Tx:**
- Multidisciplinary team approach—oncologist, radiotherapist, orthopedist
- Goals of treatment—relief of pain, ease nursing care, early mobilization, return of patient to baseline functional status
- Radiotherapy—pain relief, shrink tumor as adjunct for planned surgical excision
- Chemotherapy—directed toward primary disease, most successful as adjuvant following surgical and/or irradiative debulking of the tumor
- Surgical—includes initial biopsy, debulking of tumor to prevent or treat fractures

**Complications:** Pathologic fractures, also complications due to treatment (AVN 2° irradiation)

## 4.28 MORTON'S NEUROMA

**Etiology:** Perineural fibrosis and degeneration of the interdigital nerve 2° to entrapment and compression; most common in the 3rd web space of foot

**S/S:**
- Well-localized tenderness between metatarsal heads
- Dysesthesias in the involved web space
- +/– palpable click with compression of the metatarsal heads while pressure applied to plantar foot

**Dx:** Clinical diagnosis, confirmed with injection of lidocaine into the web space with suspected lesion

**Tx:**
- Accommodative shoes (wide toe box, low heel), metatarsal pad or bar, steroid injection into the web space
- Surgical excision for those cases that fail conservative treatment

**Complications:** Recurrence; atrophy of surrounding fat pad and rupture of collateral ligament (with steroid injections)

## 4.29 NURSEMAID'S ELBOW

**Etiology:** Radial head subluxation 2° to longitudinal traction force on extended elbow, causes a rent in the annular ligament allowing radial head to sublux

**S/S:**
- Arm held in slight flexion, forearm pronated
- Refusal to move elbow
- TTP
- Pain with any motion
- Minimal swelling early, ↑ with time

**Dx:** Clinical diagnosis; x-rays often inconclusive (due to spontaneous reduction with positioning of arm to take x-ray)

**Tx:** Closed reduction is performed by supination of forearm with pressure on radial head, +/– flexion of elbow

**Complications:** Recurrence, residual instability

## 4.30 OSTEOARTHRITIS

**Etiology:** A noninflammatory "wear-and-tear" disease of the articular surface

**S/S:** Joint pain worse with activity, better with rest; morning stiffness; joint swelling; joint deformities; HEBERDEN'S NODES; BOUCHARD'S NODES; bony enlargement; ↓ and painful ROM; crepitus; tenderness to palpation

**Dx:**
- Clinical exam will reveal high degree of suspicion, confirmed by x-rays
- X-rays—joint space narrowing, subchondral sclerosis, osteophyte formation, subchondral cysts

**Tx:**
- NSAIDs or acetaminophen for pain; intra-articular steroid injections; physical therapy; supplements (glucosamine/chondroitin) may have some benefit; viscosupplementation
- Surgery—many procedures depending on joint(s) affected

**Complications:** ↓ quality of life, chronic pain, complications of surgery (failure, infection, death)

## 4.31 PAGET'S DISEASE

**Etiology:** A disease of excessive bone destruction and disorganized remodeling; new bone is architecturally unstable, which leads to bone deformities and frequent fractures

**S/S:** Pain, usually localized to affected bone(s); FRONTAL BOSSING; anterior bowing of femur/tibia; kyphosis; deafness, tinnitus, vertigo, and cranial nerve palsies due to nerve compression by enlarged bone

**Dx:**
- X-ray—dense, coarsened trabeculae, multiple fractures, and remodeled cortices
- Bone scan—most sensitive, may show lesion before x-rays can
- Bone biopsy—to distinguish from metastatic bone disease
- Labs—↑ alkaline phosphatase level, normal calcium and phosphate

**Tx:**
- Treatment aimed at slowing osteoclastic activity—bisphosphonates; subcutaneous or nasal calcitonin
- Pain control—NSAIDs, acetaminophen
- Surgery—fracture fixation, total joint replacement, corrective osteotomies

**Complications:** Arthritis, ↑ incident of osteosarcomas

## 4.32 RHEUMATOID ARTHRITIS

**Etiology:** A chronic inflammatory state of unknown etiology characterized by synovial proliferation, cartilage destruction, and bony erosion

**S/S:** Early-morning stiffness; symmetrical joint pain and swelling, ↑ with motion, ↓ with rest; fever, malaise; SWAN–NECK DEFORMITY; BOUTONNIERE DEFORMITY; subcutaneous nodules; extra-articular manifestations (keratoconjunctivitis, scleromalacia perforans, pleuropericarditis, pulmonary nodules)

**Dx:**
- Joint fluid aspiration ≥ 2000 WBCs/μL; > 75% PMNs; absence of crystals
- Anemia of chronic disease; ↑ ESR
- 4 of 7 Dx criteria (see next card)

**Tx:**
- Conservative treatment—rest, hot baths, paraffin wax, physiotherapy
- Pain relief—NSAIDs, ASA, acetaminophen
- Medications—methotrexate, hydroxychloroquine, sulfasalazine, minocycline, gold salts, intra-articular steroids, low-dose prednisone
- TNF-α–receptor antibodies (etanercept, infliximab), IL-1 receptor antibody (anakinra)
- Surgery—reconstructive surgery for destructive arthropathy

**Complications:** Decreased life expectancy by 3–7 years; permanent joint deformities, carpal tunnel syndrome, vasculitis, pericardial effusion, atlantoaxial subluxation

## 4.33 RHEUMATOID ARTHRITIS: DIAGNOSTIC CRITERIA

**Criteria:** Diagnosis requires 4 of 7 criteria:
1. Morning stiffness lasting > 1 hr experienced for > 6 wks
2. Symmetrical joint swelling for > 6 wks
3. Must involve PIP, MCP, or wrist joint
4. More than three joints affected for > 6 wks
5. Subcutaneous nodules
6. Positive rheumatoid factor
7. X-ray evidence of joint erosion or osteopenia of hand or wrist

## 4.34 ROTATOR CUFF DISEASES

**Etiology:**
- Impingement (I)—impingement of the cuff on the acromion and overlying coracoacromial ligament
- Rotator cuff tear (RCT): may be acute or chronic, partial or complete; usually due to trauma (acute) or chronic impingement, which leads to thinning degeneration of the cuff; tear usually occurs due to microtrauma or excessive overhead use of arm

**S/S:**
- I—pain on external rotation and abduction, weakness and pain with muscle testing, ↓ AROM, normal PROM
- RCT—chronic—insidious onset of pain and weakness, progressive; acute—history of fall onto outstretched arm, immediate pain and weakness

**Dx: X-rays:**
- Normal, possible osteophyte formation on underside of acromion
- RCT sclerosis and cyst formation in greater tuberosity, osteophytes to acromion and AC joint, +/− narrowed acromiohumeral space
- MRI may show edema or frank tear to cuff tendons

**Tx:**
- Nonoperative—activity modification, NSAIDs, subacromial corticosteroid injections, stretching and strengthening
- Operative—arthroscopic subacromial decompression, débridement, +/− open or miniopen rotator cuff repair

**Complications:** Persistent pain and weakness, irreparable massive tear, DJD of the glenohumeral joint and acromioclavicular joint

## 4.35 SCOLIOSIS

**Etiology:** Idiopathic, may be infantile (birth–3 yrs), juvenile (4–10 yrs), or adolescent (> 10 yrs) based on age at onset; many other types (congenital, neuromuscular, neurofibromatosis, osteochondrodystrophy)

**S/S:** No symptoms; if pain is presenting symptom work up for other etiologies (osteoid osteoma, tethered cord); often found incidentally on school P/E or screening

**Dx:**
- Standing AP of entire thoracic and lumbar spine, curve is measured by using COBB METHOD, side bending studies assess correctability of curve
- Abnormal findings on neuro exam require further w/u with CT/MRI
- ↓ pulmonary function requires PFTs

**Tx:**
- Curve < 10°—observation
- Curve > 20°—bracing for younger patients or those who have a documented progression
- Curve > 30°—all should have braces applied
- Curve > 40°—surgical correction: posterior fusion +/− anterior release and fusion

**Complications:** Neurologic compromise, cardiopulmonary problems, infection, pseudoarthrosis, decompensation, flatback syndrome, low back pain

## 4.36  SHOULDER DISLOCATION, ANTERIOR

**Etiology:** Forced external rotation and extension of the shoulder; the most common type of dislocation (95%)

**S/S:** Severe pain, pt holds arm in position of abduction and external rotation, deformity about the shoulder (flattening to deltoid and posterior shoulder), ↑ pain with any motion

**Dx:** X-rays: AP and a lateral view of the glenohumeral joint (scapular Y or axillary lateral)

**Tx:** Closed reduction in ED or OR will reduce most dislocations; open reduction is rarely required. If reduction is stable after reduction, place arm in shoulder immobilizer

**Complications:** Recurrent instability, rotator cuff tear, brachial plexus injury, axillary nerve injury, fractures, glenoid labral tears

## 4.37  SHOULDER DISLOCATION, POSTERIOR

**Etiology:** Posteriorly directed blow to the front of the shoulder or force directed toward the abducted, flexed, and internally rotated humerus; most commonly seen with seizures or electrical shock

**S/S:** Pain, ↓ ROM, prominence to the posterior aspect of the shoulder with flattening anteriorly; arm held in abducted and internally rotated position

**Dx:** X-rays—AP may appear normal, must have axillary lateral or scapular Y view to Dx

**Tx:** Closed reduction in ED or rarely open reduction may be necessary; if reduction is stable, may place arm in shoulder immobilizer; if unstable, may need splinting in 20° of external rotation

**Complications:** Same as anterior shoulder dislocation

## 4.38 SLIPPED CAPITAL FEMORAL EPIPHYSIS

**Etiology:** Immediate cause is mechanical, during rapid growth the physeal plate is not strong enough to hold the femoral head; hormonal imbalance has been implicated; there is a hereditary predisposition

**S/S:** Vague thigh or groin pain, may progress to knee pain, limp, ↓ ROM especially IR and abduction; onset may be acute (2° minor trauma), chronic or acute on chronic

**Dx:** X-rays—AP and frog-leg lateral will show slip

**Tx:** Requires surgical epiphysiodesis in situ, may require subsequent femoral osteotomy

**Complications:** Usually related to attempted reduction of slip; AVN, chondrolysis, DJD common in later life

## 4.39 SPINAL STENOSIS

**Etiology:** Narrowing of the spinal canal → compression of the neural elements, may be congenital, developmental, or degenerative

**S/S:**
- Insidious onset of low back pain and stiffness, pain ↑ with weather changes, mechanical in nature; usually radiates to buttocks and legs; pain ↑ with standing and walking, ↓ with lying, sitting, or bending forward
- P/E—usually normal neuromuscular exam, pain with extension of L-spine and palpation of sciatic notch/SI joint

**Dx:**
- X-ray—disk-space narrowing, facet osteoarthritis, +/− spondylolisthesis, degenerative scoliosis
- MRI—reveals degree of both central and foraminal stenosis

**Tx:**
- Conservative—PT (flexion exercises, ABD strengthening, aerobic fitness exercises), NSAIDs, +/− epidural corticosteroid injections
- Surgical—decompression (laminectomy, laminotomy, discectomy)

**Complications:** Postoperative instability, recurrent stenosis

## 4.40 SPONDYLOARTHROPATHIES

**Etiology:** Inflammatory polyarthropathies characterized by sacroiliitis and the presence of HLA-B27; includes:
- Reiter's syndrome—urethritis, conjunctivitis, and lower limb polyarthritis
- Reactive arthritis—Reiter's syndrome following infectious diarrhea or chlamydial infection
- Psoriatic arthritis
- Inflammatory bowel disease–associated arthropathy

**S/S:** Low back pain, limited spinal motion, limited chest expansion, +/− sacroiliitis, ENTHESOPATHY, iritis, KERATODERMA BLENNORRHAGICA, mucocutaneous lesions, aortic insufficiency

**Dx:**
- Labs—↑ ESR, IgA, +/− HLA-B27
- X-ray—sacroiliitis

**Tx:**
- NSAIDs are 1st line for both pain and inflammation
- PT—daily exercise program with emphasis on extension exercises
- +/− methotrexate or steroids for refractory cases
- Intra-articular steroid injections for acutely inflamed joints

**Complications:** Severe articular destruction requiring joint replacement, infections secondary to injections, pain and/or dysfunction

## 4.41 SYSTEMIC LUPUS ERYTHEMATOSUS

**Etiology:** Chronic inflammatory disease of uncertain etiology characterized by B-cell hyperreactivity, activation of complement, and T-cell defects

**S/S:**
- Malar (butterfly) or discoid (red, raised, scaly) rash, fatigue, myalgias, arthralgias, photosensitivity; seizures, cognitive dysfunction, fever, alopecia
- Arthritis—symmetrical and migratory, especially in fingers, hands, wrists, and knees
- Lymphadenopathy, edema secondary to renal disease

**Dx:** See diagnostic criteria (Card 4.42)

**Tx:**
- Avoid sun exposure
- NSAIDs (arthralgias, myalgias, fever); hydroxychloroquine (rash)
- Glucocorticoids, cytotoxic drugs (severe disease or complications)
- Warfarin (anticoagulation); IVIG (acute thrombocytopenia, hemolytic anemia)

**Complications:** Tendon disease and rupture, avascular necrosis, thrombosis, vasculitis, glomerulonephritis, pericarditis, pleural effusions, pneumonitis, thromboembolic events

## 4.42 SYSTEMIC LUPUS ERYTHEMATOSUS: DIAGNOSTIC CRITERIA

**Criteria:** Must have 4 of the following 11 criteria:

1. Malar rash
2. Discoid rash
3. Photosensitivity
4. Oral ulcers
5. Arthritis
6. Serositis
7. Renal disorders (proteinuria or casts)
8. Neurologic disorders (seizures or psychosis)
9. Hematologic disorders (hemolytic anemia, leukopenia, lymphophenia, thrombocytopenia)
10. Immunologic disorders (positive LE cell preparation, anti-DNA antibody, anti-Sm antibody, false-positive serologic test for syphilis)
11. Abnormal titer of ANA

## 4.43 VOLKMANN'S ISCHEMIC CONTRACTURE

**Etiology:** Sequela of a brachial artery insult at the elbow, most commonly associated with supracondylar humeral fractures in children; not seen as often today; 2° to better treatment options now available for supracondylar humeral fractures

**S/S:**
- Loss of function to muscles in the forearm compartment and intrinsic muscles; sensation may be intact
- In later stages, muscle atrophy and fibrosis lead to contracture of the hand and ↓ ROM to wrist and elbow

**Dx:** Clinical diagnosis, suspicion ↑ with history of compartment syndrome to arm or forearm

**Tx:** Once contracture occurs, there is no treatment; best option is to identify and treat compartment syndrome or vascular injury before permanent damage occurs

**Complications:** Complete loss of function to the extremity

# CHAPTER 5

# Eyes, Ears, Nose, and Throat

## 5.1 ACOUSTIC NEUROMA

**Etiology:** Schwannoma of the vestibular nerve

**S/S:** Unilateral hearing loss, poor speech discrimination, tinnitus, vestibular symptoms (unsteadiness and imbalance)

**Dx:** MRI with gadolinium of cerebellopontine angle

**Tx:** Surgical excision of lesion or local radiation

**Complications:** Permanent loss of hearing

## 5.2 AMBLYOPIA

**Etiology:** ↓ visual acuity that is uncorrectable with lenses, no detectable anatomic defect in the eye or visual pathways; many causes (alcohol, drug toxicity, neurogenic, strabismus, tobacco, nutritional)

**S/S:** Visual impairment: blurring, spots before eyes, field defects, blindness

**Dx:** Visual acuity testing at early age (by age 4 years)

**Tx:** Correct refractive error, patch good eye, cataract or lid surgery to correct occlusion, strabismus surgery to realign eyes

**Complications:** Permanent loss of vision

## 5.3 APHTHOUS STOMATITIS

**Etiology:** Infection, trauma, dryness, irritants, toxic agents, hypersensitivity or autoimmune conditions

**S/S:** Flat, round ulcerations with yellow fibrinoid center and red halo; may last up to a week; tend to be recurrent; occur on unkeratinized mucosa, not keratinized epithelia

**Dx:**
- Clinical diagnosis
- Direct smears and cultures may disclose a pathogen
- A solitary, undiagnosed oral lesion lasting > 1 wk that does not respond to treatment must be considered malignant until proven otherwise by biopsy

**Tx:** Bland mouth rinses and hydrocortisone-antibiotic ointments encourage healing; caustics relieve pain but cause necrosis and scar tissue, thus are not recommended

**Complications:** No direct complications

## 5.4 CATARACTS

**Etiology:** Usually associated with aging, can be caused by trauma, diabetes, may be congenital

**S/S:** Increasingly blurred vision and visual distortion

**Dx:** Thorough evaluation of the eye after pupillary dilation with an ophthalmoscope or slit lamp

**Tx:** Lens extraction (intracapsular or extracapsular) and replacement of lens

**Complications:** Glaucoma, lens-induced uveitis, retinal detachment, vitreous hemorrhage, infection, epithelial downgrowth into the anterior chamber

## 5.5 CENTRAL RETINAL ARTERY OCCLUSION

**Etiology:** Embolism, thrombosis

**S/S:**
- Sudden unilateral partial to complete painless loss of vision
- Pupil sluggish to respond to light
- Pallor of the optic disk with cherry-red fovea
- Edematous macula
- Arteries are attenuated and veins are narrow, with classic "boxcar" appearance due to segmentation of the blood in the veins

**Dx:** Clinical diagnosis

**Tx:** Immediate decompression of the anterior chamber, best results if done within 30–60 min of onset

**Complications:** Blindness, infection

## 5.6 CHOLESTEATOMA

**Etiology:** An epithelial cyst that contains desquamated keratin; may be congenital or acquired 2° to chronic OM

**S/S:** Epitympanic retraction (pocket or marginal tympanic membrane perforation that exudes keratin debris)

**Dx:**
- Otoscopic exam of the ear
- X-ray—erosions to mastoid and destruction of the ossicular chain
- MRI: evidence of facial nerve or intracranial involvement (very late finding)

**Tx:** Surgical removal

**Complications:** Permanent facial nerve injury, osteomyelitis of the mastoid or ossicles, intracranial infections

## 5.7 CONJUNCTIVITIS

**Types:**
- Bacterial (B)
- Viral (V)
- Allergic (A)

**Etiology:**
- B—*Strep. pneumoniae, Staph.* spp, *Neisseria gonorrhoeae, Chlamydia trachomatis, Haemophilus influenzae*
- V—Adenovirus (most common), HSV, varicella, EBV, influenza, echovirus, coxsackievirus
- A—environmental allergens, medications

**S/S:**
- B—significant pain, purulent discharge, no papillary changes
- V—minimal pain, no visual changes, watery discharge, no papillary changes, +/− preauricular adenopathy
- A—moderate to severe itching, foreign-body sensation, dryness, tearing, marked edema of conjunctivae

**Dx:**
- B—C&S of discharge
- V&A—clinical diagnosis based on H&P

**Tx:**
- B—topical polysporin, erythromycin, quinolones
- V—self-limiting, +/− local sulfonamide therapy to prevent 2° bacterial infection
- A—antihistamine, mast cell stabilizer or steroid drops

**Complications:**
- B—corneal scarring, entropion
- V—none
- A—refractory ulceration, steroid-induced cataracts, glaucoma

## 5.8 EPIGLOTTITIS

**Etiology:** *H. influenzae* type B

**S/S:** Inspiratory stridor, drooling, high fever, dysphagia, neck pain, acute airway obstruction

**Dx:**
- Clinical diagnosis—examine airway in OR, be prepared to intubate or perform tracheostomy if airway obstruction occurs
- X-ray: "THUMB SIGN"

**Tx:** Immediate airway intubation, IV antibiotics, hydration

**Complications:** Asphyxiation

## 5.9 EPISTAXIS

**Etiology:**
- Children—trauma
- Adults—rhinitis, nasal mucosa dryness, septal deviation and bone spurs, ETOH, antiplatelet medications, cocaine abuse, chronic HTN, bleeding diathesis
- Most common site of bleed—Kiesselbach's plexus (anterior nasal septum)
- Posterior bleeds occur most common in elderly

**S/S:** Brisk bright red bleeding from the nose, usually unilateral involvement

**Dx:** Direct visualization of nares with nasoscope

**Tx:**
- Direct pressure, vasoconstrictors, anterior packing
- Posterior bleeding requires posterior packing, admit to hospital to monitor airway and oxygen saturation
- Persistent bleeding may require embolization of affected vessels

**Complications:** Recurrence

## 5.10A EYE TRAUMA: ABRASIONS

**Etiology:** Usually due to simple trauma to the eye, like fingernail or paper

**S/S:** Severe pain and photophobia

**Dx:** Visual acuity is assessed, cornea and conjunctiva examined with light for FB, sterile fluorescein confirms abrasion

**Tx:** Antibiotic ointment, firm bandage to prevent movement of lid, pt rests for 24 hr with fellow eye closed; reevaluate the next day and remove dressing

**Complications:** When recurrent, corneal erosion

(continued)

## 5.10B EYE TRAUMA: BURNS

**Etiology:** Chemicals are the most common cause

**S/S:** Severe pain with history of splash to eye

**Dx:** By history and P/E

**Tx:**
- DO NOT attempt to neutralize; copious amounts of saline in irrigation is best initial treatment
- Carefully examine and remove any particulate matter from eye
- Dilate pupil, prophylactic topical antibiotics should be initiated
- Severe burns require topical corticosteroids and topical and systemic vitamin C

**Complications:** Secondary bacterial infection, mucus deficiency, corneal scarring, tear duct obstruction, conjunctival scarring, symblepharon

## 5.10C EYE TRAUMA: FOREIGN BODIES

**Etiology:** May be under the lid or on the cornea; rarely may be found intraocular with penetrating trauma

**S/S:** Feeling of something in the eye

**Dx:** After recording visual acuity, apply local anesthetic and examine eye with flashlight, using oblique illumination

**Tx:**
- Remove foreign body with saline-soaked cotton-tipped applicator
- Apply antibiotic ointment once material has been removed
- Steel FB should have débridement of tissue stained by rust

**Complications:** Secondary bacterial infection

## 5.10D EYE TRAUMA: LACERATIONS

**Etiology:** May involve lid, conjunctiva, cornea, or sclera

**S/S:** History of trauma, visible laceration

**Tx:**
- When cornea or sclera is lacerated, eye must not be manipulated; patch loosely and cover both eyes; have patient lie quietly and refer immediately to ophthalmologist
- For conjunctival lacerations, sutures are not usually needed; apply sulfonamides or other antibiotic until the eye is healed

**Complications:** Extrusion of intraocular contents (corneal/scleral lacerations)

## 5.11 GLAUCOMA, ACUTE ANGLE CLOSURE

**Etiology:** Occurs in only patients with an anatomically narrow anterior chamber → sudden ↑ in intraocular pressure 2° to a block of the anterior chamber angle cuts off all aqueous outflow; may also occur due to sudden ↑ in the volume of the posterior chamber 2° to subchoroidal hemorrhage, swollen lens, ciliary block, or therapeutic procedures

**S/S:** Sudden onset of severe pain, blurry vision, rainbow-colored halo around lights, N/V; P/E—eye is red, cornea steamy, pupil moderately dilated and nonreactive to light

**Dx:** Tonometry—↑ intraocular pressure

**Tx:**
- Medical—oral glycerin (1 mL/kg of body weight in cold 50% solution mixed with chilled lemon juice); if patient unable to take glycerin or not responsive to it → mannitol 20% IV +/− pilocarpine 2%
- Surgical—indicated for all cases, even if medical treatment successful → laser iridectomy

**Complications:** Formation of peripheral anterior synechiae, cataract formation, atrophy of retinal and optic nerve, absolute glaucoma (stony-hard eyeball, sightless and usually painful)

## 5.12 GLAUCOMA, PRIMARY OPEN ANGLE

**Etiology:** A familial, genetically determined disorder caused by ↑ intraocular pressure 2° to interference with aqueous outflow and/or increased aqueous production

**S/S:**
- Gradual loss of peripheral vision over time = tunnel vision; persistent ↑ intraocular pressure, +/− "halos" around lights or photophobia
- P/E—Disk margin thins, cup → wider and deeper, large vessels are displaced and affected area of the disk becomes atrophic

**Dx:** Tonometry, ophthalmoscopic exam of the optic nerve, and testing of central visual field make up the "gold standard" for diagnosis and monitoring

**Tx:**
- Medical—miotics; laser trabeculoplasty—initial ↓ in pressure usually lasts months to years
- Surgical—trephine, sclerectomy, thermal sclerostomy

**Complication:** Blindness

## 5.13 HEARING LOSS

**Types:**
- Conductive—due to dysfunction of the external or middle ear; 4 mechanisms: obstruction, mass loading, stiffness effect, and discontinuity; usually correctable with medical or surgical treatment
- Sensory—due to deterioration of the cochlea, usually 2° to loss of hair cells; not correctable, may be prevented or stabilized
- Neural—due to lesions involving the eighth nerve, auditory nuclei, ascending tracts, or auditory cortex; least common clinically recognized cause of hearing loss; examples: acoustic neuroma, multiple sclerosis, cerebrovascular disease

**Evaluation:** Must evaluate in a quiet room; evaluate by speaking in a soft whisper, a normal spoken voice, or a shout; have patient repeat aloud the words spoken: WEBER TEST, RINNE TEST, formal audiometric studies

**Classifications:**
- Mild loss: threshold of 20–40 dB (soft spoken voice)
- Moderate loss: threshold of 40–60 dB (normal spoken voice)
- Severe loss: threshold of 60–80 dB (loud spoken voice)
- Profound loss: threshold of 80 dB (shout)

## 5.14 KEITH-WAGNER-BARKER CLASSIFICATION: RETINAL FINDINGS

**Classification:** Means of quantifying retinal changes in hypertension:

- Stage I—minimal narrowing or sclerosis of arterioles; corresponds with clinical classification of essential hypertension
- Stage II—copper-wire appearance of vessels, localized and generalized narrowing of arterioles, A-V nicking, scattered tiny round or flame-shaped hemorrhages, +/− vascular occlusion; corresponds with clinical classification of essential hypertension
- Stage III—"angiospastic retinopathy" = localized arteriolar spasm, hemorrhages, exudates, cotton-wool patches, retinal edema; corresponds with clinical classification of malignant hypertensive retinopathy
- Stage IV—same as stage III + optic disk swelling; corresponds with clinical classification of malignant hypertensive retinopathy

## 5.15 MACULAR DEGENERATION

**Types:**
- Atrophic (dry)—characterized by variable degrees of atrophy and degeneration of the outer retina, retinal pigment epithelium, Bruch's membrane, and choriocapillaris
- Exudative (wet)—serous fluid or blood from the choroids leaks through small defects in the collagenous membrane—focal dome-shaped elevation of the pigment epithelium

**Etiology:** Exact cause unknown

**Risk Factors:** Age > 50, white, female, family history and past or current history of cigarette smoking

**S/S:**
- Dry—progressive loss of central vision; ophthalmoscopic exam shows <u>DRUSEN</u>, clumps of pigment irregularly interspersed with depigmented areas of atrophy
- Wet—a rapid ↓ in vision may occur within days; ophthalmoscopic exam shows +/−geographic area of depigmentation at the involved site, subretinal hemorrhage, sub- and intraretinal hard exudate, overlying detachments of the retinal pigment epithelium and sensory retina, +/− "dirty gray" subretinal membrane with or without a surrounding pigmentary ring

**Dx:** Fluorescein angiography
- Dry—irregular patterns of retinal pigment epithelial hyperplasia and thinning
- Wet—neovascularization: lacy, delicate vascular networks that leak dye profusely

**Tx:**
- Dry—none
- Wet—laser photocoagulation

**Complications:** Progression from dry to wet, blindness

## 5.16 OPTIC NEURITIS

**Etiology:** Idiopathic, may be associated with demyelinating diseases (M.S.)

**S/S:**
- Unilateral visual loss, develops suddenly and progresses for a few days before reaching a plateau, then resolves → total process takes 6–8 weeks
- P/E—Pain with eye motion, central visual loss, ↓ color vision, optic disk swollen, +/− flame-shaped peripapillary hemorrhages

**Dx:**
- CSF—oligoclonal bands
- Evoked potentials
- MRI—multiple white matter lesions in the brain

**Tx:** Observation, +/− IV steroids

**Complications:** Permanent ↓ visual acuity

## 5.17 ORAL CANDIDIASIS

**Etiology:** Overgrowth of *Candida* species

**Risk Factors:** Dentures, debilitating or acute severe illness, broad-spectrum antibiotics, chemotherapy, corticosteroids, HIV/AIDS

**S/S:** Curd-like patches of creamy material in the oral cavity, surrounding mucosa is erythematous and base easily bleeds when surface scraped off; pain, halitosis, dysgeusia

**Dx:** Clinical diagnosis; confirmed by wet prep with potassium hydroxide

**Tx:** "Swish and swallow": nystatin 500,000 U 3× daily for 5–7 days

**Complications:** Chronic angular cheilitis

## 5.18  OTITIS EXTERNA

**Etiology:** Gram-negative rods are most common pathogens

**S/S:** Otalgia, pruritus, purulent discharge, erythema and edema of ear canal, pain on manipulation of auricle

**Dx:** Clinical diagnosis

**Tx:** Protect ear canal from additional moisture, avoid scratching, otic drops with aminoglycoside antibiotics and corticosteroids

**Complications:** Chronic infection (malignant external otitis), osteomyelitis, cranial nerve palsy, brain infection

## 5.19  OTITIS MEDIA, ACUTE

**Etiology:** Inflammation of the middle ear space, precipitated by viral URI or bacterial infection; common pathogens: *Strep. pneumoniae, H. influenzae, Moraxella catarrhalis*

**S/S:** Pain, erythema to TM, ↓ mobility of TM, bloody/purulent drainage, otalgia, aural pressure, ↓ hearing, fever, TM bulging or rupture

**Dx:** Clinical diagnosis

**Tx:** Antibiotics: amoxicillin or azithromycin (1st line), augmented penicillins or Bactrim (2nd line)

**Complications:** Mastoiditis, petrositis, labyrinthitis, facial paralysis, hearing loss, meningitis, lateral sinus thrombosis, subperiosteal abscess, intracranial subdural abscess

## 5.20 PERITONSILLAR ABSCESS

**Etiology:** Infection penetrating tonsillar capsule due to tonsillar infection, dental caries, or allergies

**S/S:** Fever, drooling, odynophagia, trismus, muffled voice, displacement of soft palate and uvula

**Dx:** Clinical diagnosis; cultures and sensitivities of purulent discharge to direct antibiotic coverage

**Tx:** Stabilize airway, immediate I&D with tonsillectomy, IV antibiotics followed by oral antibiotics

**Complications:** Extension to retropharyngeal, deep neck, or posterior mediastinal spaces; aspiration of pus into lungs → pneumonia

## 5.21 RETINAL DETACHMENT

**Etiology:** Cataract surgery, myopia, trauma, proliferative retinopathy of DM, severe uveitis

**S/S:** Painless blurred vision with "a curtain drawn over my eye" description, +/− floaters, flashes of light

**Dx:** Measure visual acuity, ophthalmoscopic exam with retina seen hanging in the vitreous like a gray cloud

**Tx:** Surgical repair as soon as possible

**Complications:** Repeated surgery needed, persistent detachment, blindness if macula is detached

## 5.22 RHINITIS

**Types:**
- Allergic (A)
- Vasomotor (V)

**Etiology:**
- A—pollens, grasses, ragweed, dust, and household mites are most common allergens
- V—intermittent rhinitis of unknown etiology, aggravated by dry atmosphere

**S/S:**
- A—sneezing, rhinorrhea, eye irritation, pruritus, erythema, excessive tearing
- V—sneezing, watery rhinorrhea, periods of remission and exacerbation

**Dx:** Clinical diagnosis; A—specific allergens may be tested for by either skin testing or serum RAST tests if desensitization is desired

**Tx:**
- A—symptomatic treatment with OTC antihistamines and decongestants; intranasal corticosteroids or cromolyn; maintenance of allergen-free environment
- V—empirical treatment: humidified air, systemic sympathomimetic amines

**Complications:** A—nasal polyps

## 5.23 SINUSITIS

**Etiology:** Undrained collection of pus within a sinus, usually 2° to edematous mucosa; obstruction of a sinus drainage tract

**S/S:**
- Same as rhinitis but also with pain over the affected sinus
- Maxillary—pain and pressure over the cheek, +/− pain to upper teeth
- Ethmoiditis—pain and pressure over the high lateral wall of the nose +/− radiation to the orbit
- Sphenoid—headache "in the middle of the head," +/− CN VI palsy;
- Frontal—pain and tenderness to the forehead in the area just below the medial end of the eyebrow

**Dx:**
- Clinical diagnosis, confirmed by x-ray or CT of sinuses
- Cultures of purulent drainage should be taken when untypical pathogens are suspected
- Transillumination can be done but is not helpful in most cases due to anatomic variations

**Tx:** Decongestants—oral or intranasal sprays; antibiotics—oral for most cases; if unresponsive within 2 weeks, IV should be considered

**Complications:** Chronic empyema, osteomyelitis, mucocele, hematogenous spread of infection (cavernous sinus thrombosis or meningitis), and direct extension of infection (epidural and intraparenchymal brain abscesses)

## 5.24 VERTIGO

**Types:**
- Ménière's syndrome
- Labyrinthitis (L)
- Positional vertigo (PV)

**Etiology:**
- MS—distention of the lymphatic compartment of the inner ear
- L—unknown, often follows URI
- PV—changes in head position causing vertigo, possibly due to vertebrobasilar insufficiency, dysfunction of the C-spine, or head trauma

**S/S:**
- MS—aural fullness, sensorineural hearing loss, tinnitus, episodic vertigo lasting hours
- L—severe vertigo lasting days to weeks, hearing loss, tinnitus; classic: rapid head movement causing transient vertigo
- PV—sudden, episodic vertigo with rapid head movements, lasts less than 1 minute, no hearing ↓

**Dx:** CT or MRI of the brain; persistent vertigo requires audiologic evaluation, caloric stimulation, electronystagmography, and brainstem auditory evoked potential studies

**Tx:**
- MS—low-sodium diet, diuretics, surgical decompression of end lymphatic sac
- L—meclizine or benzodiazepines PRN
- PV—meclizine PRN, constant repetition of the positional change leads to habituation

**Complications:** None

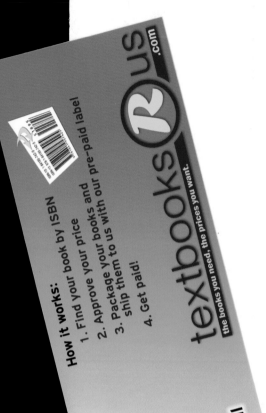
CHAPTER 6

# Reproductive System

## 6.1  ABRUPTIO PLACENTAE

**Etiology:** Premature separation of placenta

**Risk Factors:** Previous placental abruption, preeclampsia or HTN, multiparity, trauma, substance abuse (tobacco, alcohol, amphetamines, cocaine)

**S/S:** Painful 3rd trimester vaginal bleeding, abdominal pain, uterine contractions, tenderness, fetal distress

**Dx:** Contractions, bleeding; US may show retroplacental clot with large abruptions but may be normal with small ones

**Tx:**
- Observation for stable preterm fetus
- Tocolytics, fetal monitoring, delivery of fetus for moderate to severe abruption
- Give Rh immune globulin to all Rh-negative patients

**Complications:**
- Fetal—fetal distress, fetal death, preterm delivery
- Maternal—hemorrhagic shock, coagulopathy, renal failure

## 6.2  ADENOMYOSIS

**Etiology:** A type of endometriosis; endometrial tissue is found within the myometrium → hypertrophy and hyperplasia

**S/S:** Asymptomatic in 20%, dysmenorrhea in 30%, menorrhagia in 50%; globally enlarged uterus

**Dx:**
- Bimanual exam—soft, symmetrically enlarged uterus
- Biopsy, MRI

**Tx:**
- NSAIDs for symptomatic relief
- Definitive treatment is hysterectomy

**Complications:** Sterility

## 6.3 BENIGN PROSTATIC HYPERTROPHY

**Etiology:** An enlargement of the prostate not caused by cancer, infection, or other pathologic processes

**S/S:** Urinary hesitancy, urinary urgency; nocturia; sensation of incomplete emptying; poor urinary stream; urinary dribbling; dysuria; enlarged prostate on DRE (without nodules or tenderness)

**Dx:**
- UA—should be normal
- Labs—PSA; creatinine
- Postvoid residual—determine degree of incomplete emptying

**Tx:**
- Usually start with medications; surgery is reserved for severe or unresponsive cases
- Medical therapy—α-adrenergic blocking agents; 5-α-reductase enzyme inhibitor agents
- Surgical therapy—TURP; balloon dilatation of the prostate

**Complications:** Progressive obstruction, UTIs

## 6.4 BREAST CARCINOMA

**Risk Factors:** Previous breast cancer, family history, *BRCA* gene mutations, ↑ estrogens (early menarche, late menopause, nulliparity, OCP use, hormone replacement therapy, obesity)

**S/S:** Asymptomatic breast mass; bloody discharge; unilateral discharge; asymmetry of breasts; skin changes and dimpling of skin; nipple retraction; lymphadenopathy

**Dx:**
- Mammography—annually over age 40
- US—for symptomatic patients, distinguishes between solid or cystic lesions
- MRI—to evaluate questionable lesions
- Fine needle aspiration—to drain cystic lesions, solid lesions obtain sample for cytologic exam
- Core-needle biopsy—for large lesion, better yield than FNA
- Excisional biopsy is definitive

**Tx:**
- Breast conservation surgery—lumpectomy, axillary lymphadenectomy, postoperative radiation
- Modified radical mastectomy
- Adjuvant therapy if + lymph nodes: tamoxifen for 2–5 years (if estrogen/progesterone receptors are present on tumor cells); multidrug chemotherapy for 4–6 months; radiation for local treatment; ovarian ablation in premenopausal patients

**Complications:** Criteria for inoperability: extensive edema of breast/arm, satellite nodules, inflammatory carcinoma, parasternal tumor, supraclavicular or distant metastases

## 6.5  CERVICAL CARCINOMA

**Etiology:** Squamous cell: 80% of all cases, adenosquamous: 15%, remaining cases are rare histologies

**Risk Factors:** HPV infection, early onset of sexual activity, multiple partners, smoking, STDs, high parity, immunosuppression, low socioeconomic status, history of vulvar or vaginal squamous dysplasia

**S/S:**
- Abnormal bleeding, watery, blood-tinged, mucoid, purulent, or malodorous discharge
- Late signs—referred pain to flank/leg, dysuria, hematuria, rectal bleeding, obstipation, persistent edema of LE, massive hemorrhage, uremia

**Dx:**
- Pap smear, colposcopy with biopsy, +/− cone biopsy
- CT and MRI valuable for treatment planning
- Lab: CBC, BUN/creatinine, LFTs

**Tx:** Depends on stage (Card 6.6); adjuvant postoperative radiation with ↑ risk for recurrence

**Complications:** Recurrence, metastases

## 6.6  CERVICAL CARCINOMA: STAGING

**Stage 0:** Carcinoma in situ

**Stage I:** Confined to cervix
- Ia—microscopic
- Ib—visible lesions

**Stage II:** Involves superior 2/3 of the vagina, infiltrates parametria but not the side wall

**Stage III:** Involves lower 1/3 of vagina or extends to the pelvic wall +/− hydronephrosis or nonfunctioning kidney

**Stage IV:** Extends beyond pelvis, involves mucosa of bladder or rectum

**Tx:**
- Stage 0—surgical excision, laser ablation, topical 5-RU
- Stage Ia—simple hysterectomy
- Stage Ia–II—radical hysterectomy and pelvic lymphadenectomy, or whole-pelvis radiotherapy
- Stage Ib–IV—radiation therapy plus cisplatin-based chemotherapy

## 6.7  ECTOPIC PREGNANCY

**Etiology:** Implantation of zygote outside the endometrial cavity due to tubal factors, zygote abnormalities, ovarian factors, exogenous hormones, tubal aberration, IUD use, in vitro fertilization

**Risk Factors:** *Chlamydia trachomatis* infection, prior ectopic pregnancy, tobacco use, assisted reproductive technologies, PID or STDs, prior abdominal/pelvic/tubal surgeries, endometriosis

**S/S:**
- Classic triad—missed period, irregular vaginal bleeding and lower ABD pain
- Hallmark—sudden severe, unilateral abdominal pain, +/− radiation to shoulder, ABD TTP
- Rupture—syncope, shock, +/− rebound tenderness

**Dx:** Labs: CBC, β-hCG level; US will show most

**Tx:**
- Unstable—resuscitation and immediate exploratory laparotomy
- Stable—methotrexate if unruptured and mass < 3.5 cm; exploratory laparoscopy +/− salpingostomy or salpingectomy; monitor β-hCG levels weekly until no longer detected

**Complications:** Recurrent ectopic pregnancy, possible fertility problems later in life

## 6.8  ENDOMETRIOSIS

**Etiology:** The presence of functioning endometrial tissue outside the uterus

**S/S:**
- Triad of cyclic pelvic pain, dyspareunia (deep), and infertility
- Dysmenorrhea, abnormal menses, dysuria or hematuria, constipation, diarrhea, bowel frequency and/or painful defecation; suprapubic tenderness; painful nodules of uterosacral ligaments, fixed uterus; induration of cul-de-sac

**Dx:** Laparoscopy is "gold standard"; urinalysis, β-hCG; US

**Tx:** Depends on level of symptoms and desire for present and future fertility; NSAIDs (for perimenstrual symptoms), oral contraceptives, danazol and Gn-RH agonists, laparoscopic ablation of ectopic endometrial tissue, total abdominal hysterectomy (+/− bilateral salpingo-oophorectomy)

**Complications:** Recurrence; infertility

## 6.9  ERECTILE DYSFUNCTION

**Etiology:** The inability to achieve and maintain erection sufficient to perform satisfactory sexual intercourse; may be situational (specific times, places, partner) or vascular in origin

**S/S:** Inability to obtain or maintain an adequate erection; may be occasional or constant

**Dx:**
- CBC, RFT, LFT, electrolytes, TSH, free testosterone, LH/FSH, prolactin
- UA
- Screen for depression
- DHEA-S

**Tx:**
- Avoid alcohol and drugs; behavioral therapy/support
- Sildenafil (Viagra) or other medication
- Vacuum constriction of penis
- Penile prostaglandin injections
- Penile prosthesis
- Penile surgery

**Complications:** None

## 6.10  HORMONE REPLACEMENT THERAPY

**Indications:** Menopausal symptoms, osteoporosis and fracture prevention

**Side Effects:** Vaginal bleeding, migraines, breast discomfort, bloating, endometriosis exacerbation

**Eligible Patients:** Menopause symptoms, osteoporosis

**Ineligible Patients:** History of DVT, cardiac disease or CVA, breast cancer, pregnancy, liver disease

**Efficacy:**
- Menopausal symptoms—within days to weeks, full effect within 8–12 weeks
- Osteoporosis prevention—effects seen in 1–2 years

**Complications:** Venous thromboembolic events, cardiac events, CVA, breast cancer, ↑ risk of uterine/endometrial cancer (less if progesterone used), gallbladder disease

## 6.11 HYDATIDIFORM MOLE

**Etiology:** An abnormal pregnancy characterized grossly by multiple grape-like vesicles filling and distending the uterus; the most common gestational trophoblastic neoplasm, considered to arise from extraembryonic trophoblasts

**S/S:**
- Abnormal uterine bleeding, usually in the first trimester
- Hallmark is passage of vesicular tissue
- Nausea and vomiting, usually excessive (10% of time severe enough to warrant hospitalization)
- Disproportionate uterine size for gestational age
- hCG level ↑ than expected for gestational age
- Preeclampsia in first trimester or early 2nd trimester (considered pathognomonic)
- +/− hyperthyroidism

**Dx:**
- β-hCG levels ↑, need specific beta subunit assay
- Transabdominal amniocentesis + amniography; when little to no fluid is obtained inject dye and characteristic honeycomb pattern is produced by the dispersion of the dye around the vesicles

**Tx:**
- Suction curettage to evacuate all molar tissue followed by gentle sharp curettage
- Blood loss is usually moderate (may require massive transfusions)
- Prophylactic chemotherapy consisting of dactinomycin for large uteri or high risk for failure of follow-up
- Must have close follow-up for blood tests and gyn exams for a minimum of 1 year

**Complications:** Trophoblastic deportations, massive fatal pulmonary emboli, malignant disease (up to 15%)

## 6.12 MASTITIS

**Etiology:** Bacterial cellulitis of the interlobular connective tissue of the breast and mammary glands

**Risk Factors:** Maternal fatigue, poor nursing technique, nipple trauma, epidemic *Staphylococcus aureus*

**S/S:** Fever, localized erythema, tenderness, induration, ↑ tactile temp of the breast, malaise, nausea, +/− fluctuance (if abscess forms)

**Dx:** Clinical diagnosis; US to rule out abscess

**Tx:** Assess nursing technique, antibiotics, moist heat, nipple hygiene

**Complications:** Abscess formation; chronic, relapsing infection requires surgical excision of subareolar duct complex

## 6.13 MENOPAUSE

**Two Stages:**
1. Perimenopause (Peri): begins 2–8 years before menopause, lasts 1 year after last period
2. Menopause: permanent cessation of menstruation, begins 12 months after last period

**S/S:**
- Peri: DUB, sleep disturbance, hot flashes, mood lability
- Menopause: HA, ↓ libido, vaginal dryness, pruritus and dyspareunia, hot flashes

**Dx:**
- Peri—clinical diagnosis
- Menopause—serum FSH is diagnostic

**Tx:** Oral contraceptives help control some symptoms, HRT dependent on individual patient

**Complications:** Osteoporosis, DUB, slight risk ↑ cardiovascular disease and breast CA with hormone replacement therapy

## 6.14 MENSTRUAL CYCLE PHASES

**Follicular Phase:**
- Release of FSH from pituitary → ovarian follicle development; this occurs in response to withdrawal of estrogen and progesterone during luteal phase of prior menstrual cycle
- LH stimulates theca cells to divide and produce androgens
- FSH stimulates granulosa cells → ovarian follicle produces estrogen which ↑ FSH production
- Estradiol induces endometrial proliferation, prepares uterus for implantation
- Dominant follicle prevents growth of other new follicles

**Ovulation:** At midcycle, estradiol production ↑ rapidly, surge of gonadotropins LH and FSH is secreted by the hypothalamic pituitary unit in response to ↑ estrogen ↑ in LH pulse frequency and amplitude → LH surge, precedes ovulation by approximately 35–44 hr; ovulation occurs when ↑ LH levels cause follicle to rupture

**Luteal Phase:**
- After ovulation, follicle collapses → reorganizes → granulosa cells luteinize
- Progesterone maintains the endometrial lining to receive the fertilized ovum
- If fertilization does not occur, corpus luteum ↓ and progesterone levels fall → endometrial lining sloughing (menstruation)
- Lower levels of estrogen, progesterone, and inhibin → pituitary gland to ↑ gonadotropin secretion; then a new cycle of follicular recruitment begins

**Menstruation:**
- Follicular phase—endometrium is in proliferative phase and grows in response to estrogen
- Luteal phase—endometrium enters secretory phase, as it matures → prepared to accept implantation; in absence of fertilization, estrogen and progesterone levels ↓ followed by endometrial sloughing

## 6.15 NEWBORN EVALUATION

**Apgar Score:** Used to evaluate the neonate at 1 and 5 minutes after birth

| Signs | 0 | 1 | 2 |
|---|---|---|---|
| Heartbeat (bpm) | Absent | Slow (<100) | Over 100 |
| Respiratory effort | Absent | Slow, irregular | Good, crying |
| Muscle tone | Limp | Some flexion of extremities | Active motion |
| Reflex irritability | No response | Grimace | Cry or cough |
| Color | Blue or pale | Body pink, extremities blue | Completely pink |

8–10 = normal

5–7 = moderately depressed infant

0–4 = considered asphyxiated, immediate resuscitation needed

**Skin:** Evaluate for VERNIX CASEOSA, Mongolian spots, ERYTHEMA TOXICUM NEONATORUM

**Head:** Evaluate for CAPUT SUCCEDANEUM, CEPHALOHEMATOMAS, and status of the fontanelle

**Heart and Vascular System:** Note presence of any murmurs, asymmetry in pulses, cyanosis

**Further Evaluation:** Entire body must be assessed for any deformities, asymmetry, and patency of all body orifices; activity should be noted and any abnormal reflexes require further workup

## 6.16 ORAL CONTRACEPTION METHODS

**Types:** Combination hormonal methods and progestin-only methods

### Combined:
- Estrogen and progestin; may be pills, transdermal patch, vaginal ring, or injectable
- Recommended for healthy, reproductive-age women; treatment of endometriosis, dysmenorrhea, functional ovarian cysts, and other conditions
- Contraindications—history of blood clots, estrogen-dependent cancer, smoking, hypertension, hepatic adenoma or significant hepatic dysfunction
- Health benefits—regulate menses, ↓ dysmenorrhea and PMS, ↓ risk of epithelial ovarian cancer, endometrial cancer, benign breast disease; ↓ incidence of PID and ectopic pregnancy, protects against bone loss
- Side effects—spotting, HA, nausea, bloating and weight gain, hepatic adenoma, HTN, amenorrhea
- Complications—venous thromboembolism, MI and CVA, breast cancer

**Progestin Only:**
- Progestin pills, injections or implants
- Recommended for women with history of blood clots or risk factors for cardiovascular disease; must be taken at same time every day (even 3-hr difference ↓ efficacy)
- Contraindications—unreliable pill takers
- Health benefits—similar to combination methods (does not protect against bone loss)
- Side effects—irregular bleeding, amenorrhea, hot flashes, ↓ libido, vaginal dryness, hair loss, mood swings, HA, acne, weight gain
- Complications—pregnancy (usually 2° to noncompliance with pill regimen); with injections possible ↑ risk for diabetes in breast-feeding women who had gestational diabetes

## 6.17  OVARIAN CYSTS AND TUMORS

**Etiology:**
- Functional ovarian cysts—due to normal hormonal cycling
- Ovarian tumors—80% are benign; malignant transformation may be due to chronic uninterrupted ovulation

**S/S:** Asymptomatic pelvic mass; pressure or pain in lateral pelvic region; dysmenorrhea; irregular menses; N/V; urinary complaints; endocrine abnormalities; precocious puberty

**Dx:**
- Bimanual pelvic exam
- Pelvic US is often diagnostic
- +/− CA 125
- CT or MRI

**Tx:**
- Simple cysts < 3 cm—follow with PE and US; > 3 cm and < 5 cm repeat US in 1–2 mos; > 5 cm—should be excised; any ↑ in size or pain requires reevaluation; noncyclic OCP unless contraindicated
- Complex and solid cysts—refer to gynecologist
- Ovarian CA—hysterectomy, simple excision, and/or chemotherapy

**Complications:** In ovarian CA—bowel obstruction, ascites

## 6.18  PELVIC INFLAMMATORY DISEASE

**Etiology:** Ascending infection and subsequent inflammation of the upper female genital tract; pathogens: *Neisseria gonorrhoeae, C. trachomatis, Mycoplasma hominis,* group B strep

**S/S:** Lower ABD pain, cervical motion tenderness, adnexal and uterine tenderness, dyspareunia, mucopurulent cervical discharge, fever, nausea, vomiting

**Dx:**
- Labs—↑ WBCs, ESR, CRP
- Clinical diagnosis if minimal criteria met (need 3 of the following): lower ABD tenderness, cervical motion tenderness, adnexal tenderness, abnormal cervical or vaginal discharge, +/− the above lab findings

**Tx:** Antibiotics to cover all possible organisms; if not responsive to PO antibiotics within 72 hr, admit and start IV antibiotics

**Complications:** Tubal damage and adhesions, ↑ risk of ectopic pregnancy (10-fold), infertility

## 6.19 PLACENTA PREVIA

**Etiology:** Implantation of placenta near or at the cervical os, placental attachment is disrupted at the lower uterine segment due to thinning in preparation for labor

**Risk Factors:** Advanced maternal age, multiparity, multiple gestations, and previous C-section

**S/S:** Painless, bright red 3rd trimester bleeding, +/− contractions, usually no fetal distress

**Dx:** US is diagnostic

**Tx:** Bed rest, tocolytics, betamethasone, delivery by C-section when fetal lungs are mature

**Complications:** Fetal distress, fetal death, preterm birth, maternal hemorrhagic shock

## 6.20 POLYCYSTIC OVARIAN SYNDROME

**Etiology:** Androgen excess, possibly due to excess LH stimulation of ovaries

**S/S:** HAIR-AN: **H**yperandrogenism (hirsutism); **i**nsulin **r**esistance (obesity, glucose intolerance); **a**canthosis **n**igricans (velvety, raised hyperpigmented skin lesions on back of neck, axillae, and genitalia)

**Dx:**
- Labs—hyperandrogenism; TSH, DHEA-S, and free testosterone levels; glucose, $Hb_{A1c}$, FSH, and LH
- US—enlarged ovaries plus numerous cysts with characteristic "pearl necklace" appearance (not necessary for diagnosis)

**Tx:**
- Oral contraceptives to regulate menstrual cycle
- Spironolactone—↓ hirsutism
- Clomiphene citrate—induces ovulation
- Pioglitazone (Actos)—↑ insulin sensitivity, regulates menstrual cycle
- Metformin (Glucophage)—↑ insulin sensitivity, regulates menses, induces weight loss, and decreases acanthosis nigricans
- Weight loss—↑ insulin sensitivity, regulates menses, decreases lipids

**Complications:** Pregnancy, endometrial cancer (due to estrogen excess)

## 6.21 POSTPARTUM HEMORRHAGE

**Etiology:** May be early (< 24 hr) or late (> 24 hr) after delivery
- Early—uterine atony, retained placental fragments, cervical and vaginal lacerations, uterine rupture or inversion, bleeding disorders
- Late—subinvolution of the uterus, retained placental fragments, endometritis

**S/S:** Bright red bloody vaginal discharge, hypotension, tachycardia, shock, pelvic pain, atonic boggy uterus (if uterine atony)

**Dx:**
- Clinical diagnosis—visual inspection for lacerations, palpation to detect atony, digital exploration of uterus for retained placental fragments, visual inspection of placenta for missing cotyledons
- Labs—CBC to check for anemia
- PT/PTT, fibrinogen—to evaluate for DIC

**Tx:**
- Tocolytics, volume, blood and/or clotting factors
- Atony—manual massage of uterus
- Retained placenta fragments—manual removal of fragments and curettage
- Lacerations, rupture, or inversion of uterus requires surgical intervention

**Complications:** Death, pelvic infection, anemia, transfusion reactions, infertility

## 6.22 PREECLAMPSIA

**Etiology:** A syndrome of elevated blood pressure, proteinuria, and edema due to abnormal invasion of placental cells into the uterine spiral arterioles

**Risk Factors:** First pregnancy at age > 35, multifetal gestations, molar pregnancy, underlying HTN, diabetes, obesity, black race, genetics

**S/S:**
- Classic triad—BP > 140/90, edema, proteinuria
- +/− visual disturbances, HA, epigastric pain
- Severe cases—HELLP syndrome (**h**emolysis, **e**levated **L**FTs, **l**ow **p**latelets)

**Dx:**
- BP measurements on 2 separate occasions > 140/90
- Proteinuria > 300 mg/24-hr urine collection
- Severe—BP > 160 systolic or 110 diastolic on 2 occasions at least 6 hr apart; proteinuria 5+ g in 24-hr urine specimen or 3+ g on 2 random urine samples at least 4 hr apart

**Tx:**
- Definitive treatment is delivery; may be considered as first line at 38 wks of gestation
- <38 weeks—bed rest, hydralazine to ↓ B/P, IV magnesium sulfate for seizure prophylaxis
- HELLP—must be immediately delivered regardless of gestational age

**Complications:** Maternal: pulmonary edema, hepatocellular necrosis, subcapsular hemorrhage, cerebral edema or hemorrhage, retinal detachment, DIC, postoperative bleeding, delayed wound healing, abruptio placentae, recurrence in next pregnancy, possible ↑ risk of hypertension or diabetes later in life

## 6.23 PREGNANCY, NORMAL SIGNS

**Presumptive:**
- Amenorrhea, nausea and vomiting, UTI, urinary frequency and nocturia, ↑ basal body temp
- MASTODYNIA, MONTGOMERY'S TUBERCLES, colostrum secretion, SECONDARY BREASTS
- Quickening (first perception of fetal movement usually at 14–20 wks)
- CHLOASMA, LINEA NIGRA, stretch marks (late finding)

**Probable:**
- Chadwick's sign (bluish or purplish discoloration of the vagina and cervix)
- Goodell's sign (cyanosis and softening of the cervix, as early as 4 weeks)
- Ladin's sign (softening of the uterus in the anterior midline along the uterocervical junction, at around 6 weeks)
- Hegar's sign (widening of the softened area of the isthmus and compressibility of the isthmus on bimanual exam by 6–8 weeks)
- McDonald's sign (uterus becomes flexible at the uterocervical junction at about 7–8 weeks)
- Von Fernwald's sign (irregular softening of the fundus developing over the site of implantation at 4–5 weeks)
- Leukorrhea, relaxation of the joints of the pelvis, abdominal enlargement, uterine contractions, ballottement of the uterus

**Positive:**
- Fetal heart tones, palpation of the fetus, x-ray of the fetus, ultrasound examination of the fetus
- Beta-hCG levels

## 6.24 PRENATAL CARE

**Prenatal Visit Schedule:**
- Every 4 weeks until 28th week of gestation
- Every 2–3 weeks from 28–36 weeks
- Every week after 36 weeks of gestation

**Routine Visits Should Include:** BP, maternal weight, fundal height, fetal heart tones, fetal position, observation for edema, UA (protein, glucose, blood, leukocyte esterase)

**Ultrasound:** Will visualize gestational sac at 5 weeks or at β-hCG of 1,500 mIU/mL; will detect fetal heartbeat at 6 weeks or at β-hCG of 5,000–6,000 mIU/mL

**Labs:**
- Initial—CBC, blood type/screen, RPR, rubella antibody, hepatitis B surface antigen, gonorrhea and *Chlamydia,* PPD, Pap smear, UA/culture, varicella titer, HIV screening
- TRIPLE SCREEN —15–18 weeks
- Fetal survey—18–20 weeks
- Glucose tolerance test—24–28 weeks
- Group B streptococcus screen—35–37 weeks

## 6.25  PROSTATE CARCINOMA

**Etiology:** Nearly 100% are adenocarcinomas

**S/S:** Urinary symptoms—urgency, hesitancy, poor stream; hematuria; hard prostate nodule on DRE; unilateral lymphedema; weight loss; back pain with spinal metastases

**Dx:**
- Biopsy of prostate mass is diagnostic
- Screening—DRE
- PSA
- Bone pain, ↑ alkaline phosphatase or hypercalcemia can indicate bony metastases

**Tx:** Prostatectomy; radiation therapy; hormonal therapy; androgen ablation and chemotherapy for metastases

**Complications:** Postoperative infection, erectile dysfunction, urinary incontinence, retrograde ejaculation, bowel problems, radiation proctitis (side effects of treatment)

## 6.26  PROSTATITIS

**Etiology:** Inflammation without identification of causative organism is most common cause

**S/S:**
- Acute bacterial—acute febrile illness, chills, myalgias, arthralgias; rectal, perineal, or low back pain; dysuria, urgency, and frequency
- Chronic bacterial—subacute or chronic symptoms; rectal, perineal, or low back pain; dysuria, urgency, and frequency
- Nonbacterial prostatitis/prostatodynia—rectal or perineal pain; dysuria, urgency, hesitancy, nocturia, weak urinary stream, painful ejaculation, postejaculatory pain, hematospermia

**Dx:**
- UA—WBCs, culture should yield pathogen in acute and chronic prostatitis
- DRE—boggy, tender prostate; avoid in acute bacterial prostatitis to avoid bacteremic spread

**Tx:**
- Acute bacterial—fluoroquinolones; doxycycline/ampicillin; trimethoprim/sulfamethoxazole for 4–6 wks
- Chronic bacterial—fluoroquinolones; doxycycline; cephalexin for 3+ months
- Nonbacterial and prostatodynia—tetracycline, doxycycline, or erythromycin for 6–12 weeks; $\alpha_1$-adrenergic blocking agents; NSAIDs

**Complications:** Prostatic abscess

## 6.27A  SEXUALLY TRANSMITTED DISEASES

**Etiology:**

- Herpes—herpes simplex virus
- Syphilis—*Treponema pallidum*
- Chancroid—*Haemophilus ducreyi*
- Lymphogranuloma venereum—*C. trachomatis*
- Granuloma inguinale—*Calymmatobacterium granulomatis*
- Condyloma acuminatum—HPV
- Gonorrhea—*Neisseria gonorrhoeae*
- Vaginitis—*Trichomonas vaginalis*
- Cervicitis/urethritis—*N. gonorrhoeae, Chlamydia, Ureaplasma*

**S/S:**

- **Painful** genital lesions—herpes, chancroid
- **Painless** lesions—syphilis, condyloma acuminatum, granuloma inguinale, lymphogranuloma venereum
- Herpes—painful vesicles, itching and burning, +/– fever, HA
- Lymphogranuloma venereum—fever, malaise, bilateral tender inguinal adenopathy

- Chancroid—painful, deep ulcer with exudates, followed in 1–2 weeks by painful local lymphadenitis
- Vaginitis/urethritis—purulent discharge with pubic pain +/– dysuria
- Gonorrhea/*Chlamydia*—vaginal discharge (mucopurulent discharge), urethral discharge, dysuria, urgency, frequency, pelvic pain, dyspareunia, cervical motion tenderness (PID), +/– RUQ pain (gonorrhea)
- Syphilis—1° = painless ulcer; 2° = maculopapular rash on palms and soles, mucous membrane lesions, nontender adenopathy, fever, weight loss, fatigue, sore throat; 3° = gummas (subcutaneous, ulcerative lesions of skin), neurosyphilis (paresis, TABES DORSALIS, hypotonia)
- Condyloma acuminatum—venereal warts (painless, cauliflower-like growths)
- HPV—most asymptomatic (may present with postcoital vaginal bleeding; vaginal discharge; irregular vaginal bleeding; vaginal pain; bloody, malodorous discharge); cervical exam: unexplained cervical friability, cervical nodules or thickening

*(continued)*

## 6.27B  SEXUALLY TRANSMITTED DISEASES, Continued

**Dx:**

- Herpes—clinical ID of lesion, Tzanck smear, tissue culture or serology
- Syphilis—RPR, VDRL
- Chancroid—clinical diagnosis with negative herpes/syphilis workup
- Lymphogranuloma venereum—complement fixation
- Granuloma inguinale—scraping with Wright's and Giemsa stains (show Donovan bodies)
- Urethritis/cervicitis—+ *N. gonorrhoeae* culture and *Chlamydia* test
- HPV—regular Pap smears, anal smear of homosexual men to rule out anorectal CA
- Gonorrhea—+ culture testing on cervical or urethral specimens
- *Chlamydia*—direct fluorescent antibody or enzyme immunoassay

**Tx:**

- Herpes—acyclovir for severe cases; prophylactic treatment for patients with > 5 episodes per year

- Chancroid—IM ceftriaxone (single dose) or azithromycin PO (single dose)
- *Trichomonas vaginalis*—metronidazole for 7 days
- Lymphogranuloma inguinale—tetracycline or doxycycline for 21 days
- HPV—destroy or excise warts; for dysplasia cases = colposcopy
- *Chlamydia*—doxycycline for 7 days; azithromycin, single dose (if pregnant or noncompliant); erythromycin for 7 days (if pregnant)
- Gonorrhea—ciprofloxacin, single dose; ceftriaxone IM, single dose (if pregnant); cefixime, single dose (if pregnant)
- PID—ofloxacin for 14 days; metronidazole for 14 days
- Syphilis—1°, 2°, or early 3°, penicillin IM, single dose, **or** oral doxycycline for 2 weeks (PCN allergy); 3° (> 1 year), PCN IM weekly for 3 weeks **or** oral doxycycline for 4 weeks; neurosyphilis, IV PCN 10–14 days

## 6.28 TESTICULAR CARCINOMA

**Etiology:** Germ cell in origin; seminoma, embryonal cell CA, teratoma, choriocarcinoma, mixed origin

**S/S:** Scrotal mass; lymphadenopathy; painful scrotal mass with incidental testicular trauma (due to tumor bleeding)

**Dx:**
- Scrotal US
- Labs—α-fetoprotein; quantitative β-hCG; LDH
- CT scan and node examination for staging

**Tx:**
- Emergent evaluation by urologist
- Surgery—radical orchiectomy
- Chemotherapy—advanced disease or metastases
- Radiation therapy

**Complications:** Recurrences, metastases

## 6.29 UTERINE BLEEDING, DYSFUNCTIONAL

**Etiology:** Bleeding caused by factors other than pelvic anatomic abnormalities, pregnancy, bleeding disorders, endocrine disorders, or medications

**S/S:** MENORRHAGIA, METRORRHAGIA, MENOMETRORRHAGIA, POLYMENORRHEA, OLIGOMENORRHEA, AMENORRHEA, intermenstrual bleeding, postmenopausal bleeding

**Dx:**
- Diagnosis of exclusion, must adequately exclude all possible diagnoses
- Labs—β-hCG, TSH, CBC, PT/PTT/INR
- Cervical cultures
- Pelvic US
- Endometrial biopsy—mandatory for all postmenopausal bleeding, obese, or diabetic patients

**Tx:**
- Treat underlying cause if identified
- Progesterone challenge test—temporarily stop excessive bleeding or bring on bleeding in patient who is oligomenorrheic
- Oral contraceptives—regulate flow in patients who have polycystic ovarian syndrome or need contraception
- Hormone replacement therapy—may regulate flow in perimenopausal women

**Complications:** Anemia

## 6.30  UTERINE CARCINOMA

**Types:**
- Endometrial—type I, estrogen-related; type II, unrelated to estrogen/hyperplasia
- Sarcoma—rare type of uterine cancer

**Etiology:**
- Endometrial—adenocarcinoma (80%), mucinous (5%), clear cell (5%), papillary serous (4%), squamous (1%)
- Sarcoma—arises from glands and myometrium

**S/S:**
- Endometrial—abnormal uterine bleeding, pelvic pressure/pain, pyometra, hematometra, endometrial cells on Pap smear out of phase, or in postmenopausal woman
- Sarcoma—abdominal mass/pain, rapidly enlarging uterus

**Dx:**
- Endometrial biopsy, US
- Labs—CBC, BUN/creatinine, LFTs
- CXR, CT, sigmoidoscopy to evaluate for metastatic disease

**Tx:** Total abdominal hysterectomy with bilateral salpingo-oophorectomy, +/− lymph node resection; postoperative XRT (for both endometrial and sarcoma)

**Complications:** Metastatic disease, prognosis depends on stage (Card 6.31)

## 6.31  UTERINE CARCINOMA: STAGING FOR ENDOMETRIAL CARCINOMA

**Stage I:**
- A—limited to endometrium
- B—invades < 1/2 of myometrium
- C—invades > 1/2 of myometrium

**Stage II:**
- A—endocervical glandular involvement
- B—stromal invasion

**Stage III:**
- A—uterine serosa or malignant cells in peritoneal fluid
- B—vaginal involvement
- C—pelvic/paraaortic lymph nodes

**Stage IV:**
- A—invasion of bladder/bowel mucosa
- B—distant metastasis

**Prognosis:** Five-year survival
- Stage I—90%
- Stage II—75%
- Stage III—40%
- Stage IV—10%

**Uterine Sarcoma:** Poor prognosis; 5-year survival is 50% at best; if metastases present = 20%

## 6.32 UTERINE LEIOMYOMA (FIBROID)

**Etiology:** Benign smooth muscle tumor

**S/S:** Hypermenorrhea, metrorrhagia, dysmenorrhea, pain, pressure, urinary frequency and urgency, dyspareunia, infertility, spontaneous abortion; firm, irregular uterine mass

**Dx:**
- β-hCG to rule out pregnancy
- Pap smear and endometrial biopsy
- US—usually diagnostic
- Hysterosalpingography for definitive diagnosis

**Tx:**
- Depends on patient's age, parity, pregnancy status, and desire for future fertility
- Follow with periodic examinations, Pap smear, and US
- Medroxyprogesterone (Depo-Provera) to induce amenorrhea (if hypermenorrhea)
- GnRH agonist to limit growth
- Myomectomy
- Hysterectomy

**Complications:** ↑ in size with estrogen therapy or during pregnancy; infertility; spontaneous abortion

## 6.33 VAGINAL BLEEDING, ABNORMAL

**Etiology:**
- Irregular bleeding during menstrual cycle
- Menorrhagia, metrorrhagia, polymenorrhea—associated with chronic anovulation, endometrial or cervical cancer, fibroids, endometrial hyperplasia, endometrial polyps, complications of pregnancy
- Hypomenorrhea—associated with hypogonadotropic hypogonadism, atrophic endometrium, Asherman's syndrome, OCP/HRT, intrauterine adhesions, trauma
- Oligomenorrhea—associated with pregnancy and disruptions of pituitary-gonadal axis

**S/S:**
- Menorrhagia—loss of > 80 mL of blood in 1 cycle
- Metrorrhagia—bleeding between periods
- Hypomenorrhea—unusually light menses
- Polymenorrhea—frequent periods < 21 days apart
- Oligomenorrhea—periods > 35 days apart

**Dx:** Labs—serum β-hCG, prolactin, TSH, LH, FSH; Pap smear; US, +/− endometrial biopsy

**Tx:** OCPs, progestin therapy, medroxyprogesterone, removal of fibroids/polyps, D&C, hysterectomy

**Complications:** None

# CHAPTER 7

# Endocrine System

## 7.1 ACROMEGALY

**Etiology:** Due to excessive secretion of growth hormone after closure of the epiphyses, there is overgrowth of soft tissues and terminal skeletal structures

**S/S:** Doughy enlargement of the hands with spade-like fingers; large feet, jaw, face, tongue, and internal organs; wide-spaced teeth, MOLLUSCA, hoarse voice, HA, bitemporal hemianopia, lethargy, +/− diplopia, +/− diabetes mellitus, goiter, abnormal lactation; excessive sweating most reliable sign of the activity of the disease

**Dx:**
- Labs—↑ serum inorganic phosphorus, gonadotropins normal to low, hyperglycemia, resistance to insulin, ↑ serum prolactin, ↑ serum growth hormone, hypercalciuria, glycosuria
- IV TRH or LRH—↑ growth hormone and glucose fails to ↓ serum growth hormone
- CT or MRI should show pituitary tumor when present

**Tx:** Surgical removal of the hyperfunctioning tissue

**Complications:** Pressure of the tumor on surrounding structures, rupture into the brain or sinuses, diabetes, cardiac enlargement and failure, carpal tunnel syndrome, arthritis, degenerative disk disease

## 7.2 ADDISON'S DISEASE

**Etiology:** Primary adrenocortical insufficiency (cortisol and aldosterone deficiency); most commonly due to autoimmune destruction of the adrenal cortex

**S/S:** Weakness, fatigue, weight loss, abdominal pain, anorexia, N/V, hyperpigmentation of skin and mucous membranes, hypotension, and orthostatic hypotension

**Dx:**
- ACTH stimulation test is diagnostic
- Labs—hyperkalemia, hyponatremia, hypoglycemia, eosinophilia
- ECG—peaked T waves, prolonged PR interval, heart block

**Tx:** Synthetic cortisol replacement, increase dose during periods of stress, illness, surgery; aldosterone replacement; increased sodium intake

**Complications:** Adrenal crisis

## 7.3 ADRENAL CRISIS

**Etiology:** Sudden marked deprivation or insufficient supply of adrenocortical hormones; may occur due to stress, sudden withdrawal of adrenocortical hormone, 2° to bilateral adrenalectomy or sudden destruction of the pituitary gland or injury to both adrenals by trauma

**S/S:** HA, N/V, ABD pain, fatigue, +/− diarrhea, confusion or coma, fever (up to 105°F), ↓ BP, +/− cyanosis, petechiae, dehydration, lymphadenopathy

**Dx:**
- Labs—↑ eosinophil count, ↓ serum glucose and sodium, ↑ serum potassium and BUN, hypercalcemia, cortisol levels are very ↓ (blood and urine), plasma ACTH ↑↑
- ECG—↓ voltage

**Tx:** Antishock measures, hydrocortisone phosphate or hydrocortisone sodium succinate IV, start with 100 mg IV immediately then 50–100 mg every 6 hr, taper dose daily; once crisis passes, change to oral hydrocortisone reducing level to maintenance levels as needed

**Complications:** Hyperpyrexia, LOC, generalized edema, HTN, flaccid paralysis, psychotic reactions

## 7.4 ADRENAL HYPERPLASIA, CONGENITAL

**Etiology:** A complex series of rare enzymatic errors of metabolism → deficient levels of different enzymes involved in the synthesis of cortisol

**S/S:** Masculinization in females and early virilization in males, hypocortisolism, HTN

**Dx:**
- ↑ ACTH levels, plasma androgens, urinary pregnanetriol, and 17-ketosteroids
- Hallmark—↑ plasma levels of the metabolic precursor immediately before the enzymatic block (11-deoxycortisol in 11β-hydroxylase deficiency; 17-hydroxyprogesterone in 21-hydroxylase deficiency)

**Tx:** Enough glucocorticoids to suppress ACTH and reverse the metabolic abnormalities

**Complications:** Those associated with HTN; females may also have ambiguous genitalia, requiring plastic surgery to correct

## 7.5 CUSHING'S SYNDROME

**Etiology:** Hyperfunctioning of adrenal cortex, results in hypersecretion of cortisol; Cushing's **disease** is hypercortisolism due to pituitary tumor

**S/S:** Central obesity, "buffalo hump" and increased supraclavicular fat pads, moon facies, purple abdominal striae, acne, hirsutism, edema, HTN, impaired glucose tolerance, osteoporosis, muscle weakness/fatigue, oligomenorrhea/amenorrhea, impotence/loss of libido, personality changes

**Dx:**
- Labs—hyperglycemia, leukocytosis, loss of diurnal cortisol levels, ↑ 24 hr urine cortisol
- Dexamethasone suppression test

**Tx:**
- Adrenal adenoma—resection with temporary postoperative cortisol replacement
- Adrenal carcinoma—resection or symptomatic treatment (adrenal inhibitors)
- Pituitary tumor—transsphenoidal pituitary surgery (65%–90% cure rate); pituitary irradiation in children; bilateral adrenalectomy with permanent steroid replacement
- Ectopic ACTH tumors—treat underlying cause

**Complications:** CHF, CVA, MI, diabetes, osteoporotic fractures, psychotic disorders

## 7.6 DIABETES INSIPIDUS

**Types:**
- Nephrogenic (N)
- Central (C)
- Secondary (S)

**Etiology:**
- Syndrome of either decreased secretion or ineffective action of ADH; results in an inability to reabsorb water
- N—↓ action of ADH due to insensitivity of renal tubules
- C—↓ secretion of ADH from pituitary gland
- S—due to inhibition of ADH by excessive intake of fluids

**S/S:** Polyuria, urinary frequency, enuresis, nocturia, excessive thirst, dehydration

**Dx:**
- Serum hypertonicity with inappropriate urine hypotonicity
- UA—specific gravity < 1.010; osmolality < 300 mOsm/kg
- 24-hr urine > 50 mL/kg
- Water deprivation test—overnight water restriction followed by injection of ADH
- N—no ↑ in urine concentration during water restriction; no response to ADH
- C—no ↑ in urine concentration during restriction, but + response to ADH

**Tx:**
- N—thiazide diuretics and/or amiloride, low-salt diet, prostaglandin inhibitors
- C—DDAVP, chlorpropamide, +/– diuretics
- S—treat underlying cause

**Complications:** Irreversible renal damage, adrenal insufficiency, severe dehydration, death

## 7.7  DIABETES MELLITUS

**Types:**
- Type 1—IDDM (1)
- Type 2—NIDDM (2)
- Gestational (G)

**Etiology:**
- 1—destruction of insulin-producing β cells of pancreas, results in insulin deficiency
- 2—due to impaired insulin secretion, insulin resistance, and increased hepatic glucose production
- G—due to ↑ tissue resistance to insulin secondary to secretion of human placental lactogen and ↑ levels of estrogen and progesterone

**S/S:** Polyuria, polydipsia, polyphagia, fatigue, frequent infections, end-organ symptoms (retinopathy, nephropathy, atherosclerosis, autonomic neuropathy, peripheral neuropathy, hypertension)

**Dx:** Criteria for diagnosis: symptoms plus random blood glucose > 200 mg/dL **or** fasting blood glucose > 126 **or** blood glucose > 200 during oral glucose tolerance test

**Tx:** Low-sugar diet, exercise, medications (oral agents or insulin); treat any potential complications (ASA, antihypertensives, statins, heart meds)

**Complications:** Diabetic ketoacidosis, nonketotic hyperosmolar coma, hypoglycemia, end-organ disease, SYNDROME X, SOMOGYI PHENOMENON

## 7.8  DIABETIC KETOACIDOSIS

**Etiology:** Complication of hyperglucagonemia, may be due to undiagnosed diabetes mellitus, increased insulin requirements during infection, trauma, or other stress, or as a complication of insulin pump therapy; most common cause is poor patient compliance

**S/S:** Polyuria, polydipsia, marked fatigue, N/V, mental stupor that progresses to coma, evidence of dehydration, rapid deep breathing, "fruity" breath odor, +/− hypotension, tachycardia, abdominal pain

**Dx:**
- UA—glycosuria of 4+, strong ketonuria
- Labs—hyperglycemia, ketonemia, low arterial blood pH, low plasma bicarbonate

**Tx:** Prevention is best treatment; admit severe cases for IV hydration and insulin, correct electrolyte abnormalities, treat any associated infection

**Complications:** Acute MI, infarcted bowel, renal failure, death

## 7.9 GRAVES' DISEASE

**Etiology:** Autoimmune thyroid disorder in which thyrotoxicosis occurs with associated diffuse enlargement and hyperactivity of the thyroid along with the presence of antibodies against different fractions of the gland

**S/S:** Goiter, restlessness, irritability, easy fatigability, weight loss, nervousness, excess sweating and heat intolerance, muscle tremors, exophthalmos, spider angiomas, gynecomastia, tachycardia, atrial fibrillation, lymphadenopathy, splenomegaly

**Dx:** Labs = T4, radioiodine and T3 resin uptake is ↑; serum cholesterol ↓; urinary creatine ↑; lymphocytosis, thyroid-stimulating immunoglobulins +

**Tx:** Aim is to halt excessive secretion of the thyroid gland; 3 methods:
(1)  Medical therapy—thioureas, iodine, propranolol
(2)  Subtotal thyroidectomy
(3)  Radioactive iodine ablation of the gland

**Complications:**
• Ocular—exophthalmos
• Cardiac—tachycardia, CHF, atrial fibrillation
• ↓ libido, impotence, ↓ sperm count, gynecomastia
• Hypothyroidism—may be spontaneous or treatment-induced
• Complications due to treatment—drug reactions, hypoparathyroidism, laryngeal palsy

## 7.10 HYPERALDOSTERONISM

**Etiology:**
• Primary—due to adrenal causes, direct secretion of aldosterone
• Secondary—due to extra-adrenal causes that activate the renin-angiotensin-aldosterone system

**S/S:** Excess sodium reabsorption, potassium wasting (muscle weakness, tetany, fatigue, paresthesias, dilute urine), hydrogen wasting (metabolic alkalosis), HA, polyuria, polydipsia, +/− signs of advanced HTN

**Dx:**
• Labs—hypokalemia, hypernatremia, metabolic alkalosis
• Diastolic hypertension
• 1°—↑ aldosterone with ↓ renin; 2°—↑ aldosterone with ↑ renin
• ECG = LVH, signs of hypokalemia
• UA—+/− proteinuria

**Tx:** Adrenal adenoma: resection; other causes: aldosterone antagonists, sodium restriction and antihypertensives

**Complications:** Hypertension, arrhythmias

# 7.11 HYPERPARATHYROIDISM

**Etiology:**
- Primary—excess parathyroid hormone due to causes within the parathyroid gland
- Secondary—caused by overstimulation of the parathyroids due to decreased serum calcium, usually due to chronic renal failure

**S/S:** Classic presentation—"stones, bones, abdominal groans, and psychic overtones"

**Dx:**
- 1°—serum calcium > 10.5 mg/dL with ↑ PTH; serum phosphate ↓; urine levels of calcium and phosphate ↑; +/− fractures, US/CT of parathyroid may show adenoma
- 2°—↓ serum calcium with ↑ PTH; RFT may indicate renal failure
- Pseudohyperparathyroidism—↑ serum calcium and ↑ PTHrP; +/− malignancy on studies of lung, pancreas, breast

**Tx:**
- 1°—alendronate/pamidronate; estrogen therapy; oral phosphate; ↑ fluid intake; parathyroidectomy is definitive
- 2°—correct renal failure; phosphate-binding antacids; calcium and vitamin D supplementation; calcium-rich dialysis; alendronate/pamidronate; parathyroidectomy
- Pseudo—IV pamidronate; treat underlying cancer

**Complications:** Postoperative hypocalcemia, intraoperative damage to nearby nerves

# 7.12 HYPERPITUITARISM

**Etiology:** Most common cause is pituitary adenoma—↑ GH means acromegaly; ↑ ACTH means Cushing's disease; ↑ prolactin means galactorrhea

**S/S:**
- GH—HA, swelling of hands and feet, coarse facial features, moist skin, perspiration, macroglossia, HTN, prognathism, arthritis, enlarged organs, hyperglycemia, menstrual irregularities
- Prolactin—galactorrhea, amenorrhea, HA, ↓ libido, hot flashes
- ACTH—Cushing's disease

**Dx:** Plasma growth hormone level; plasma prolactin levels; CT/MRI of head with contrast to visualize tumor

**Tx:**
- Pituitary adenoma—transsphenoidal resection, radiation is second-line therapy
- Prolactin adenoma—bromocriptine
- Acromegaly—somatostatin, dopamine agonists (inhibits GH)

## 7.13 HYPOPITUITARISM

**Etiology:** Panhypopituitarism or selective hyposecretion of specific pituitary hormone(s)

**S/S:**
- LH/FSH—amenorrhea, infertility, impotence, testicular atrophy
- TSH—hypothyroidism
- ACTH—hypoadrenalism
- GH—somatostatin deficiency syndrome
- Visual field defects due to compression of the optic chiasm by tumor

**Dx:**
- CT/MRI skull with contrast to visualize tumor
- Labs—free T4; TRH, GnRH
- Insulin tolerance test

**Tx:** Resection of adenoma, hormone replacement

**Complications:** Due to patient's inability to cope with minor stressful situations (fever, shock, coma, death)

## 7.14 HYPERTHYROIDISM

**Etiology:** Oversecretion of thyroid hormone due to nodular hyperplasia of thyroid, damage to thyroid, or diffuse over-production of thyroid hormone; may be primary (dysfunction of the thyroid gland itself) or secondary (overstimulation of the thyroid gland by excess TSH production)

**S/S:** Heat intolerance, sweating, hyperactivity, irritability, nervousness, weight loss, diarrhea, weakness, fatigue, tremor, tachycardia, palpitations, atrial fibrillation, enlarged thyroid/goiter, neck pain, lid lag/lid retraction, gynecomastia, loss of libido, menstrual irregularities

**Dx:**
- TFTs—↑ free T4, total T4, and T3; 1°—↑ T4 with ↓ TSH; 2°—normal or ↑ T4 with ↑ TSH
- Radionucleotide thyroid scan—↓ uptake means damage of thyroid or thyroid hormone ingestion
- ECG—atrial fibrillation or sinus tachycardia

**Tx:** Thyroid adenoma—radioactive iodine to ablate thyroid, antithyroid drugs; de Quervain's thyroiditis—NSAIDs, beta blockers, prednisone

**Complications:** Thyroid storm, arrhythmias, death

## 7.15 HYPOTHYROIDISM

**Etiology:** Decreased production of thyroid hormone due to Hashimoto's disease, postpartum thyroiditis, drugs, pituitary dysfunction, congenital dysplasia of the thyroid, may be 1° or 2°

**S/S:** Dry skin, coarse hair, +/− hair loss, hoarseness, weakness, dyspnea, cold intolerance, lethargy, fatigue, poor appetite, +/− weight gain, constipation, hearing loss, paresthesias, bradycardia, menstrual irregularities, delayed DTRs, goiter, myxedema, memory loss, poor concentration, +/− thyroid gland nodules or tenderness to palpation

**Dx:**
- TFTs—1°—↓ T4 with ↑ TSH; 2°—↓ T4 with low/normal TSH
- Labs—anemia, ↑ CPK, cholesterol and triglycerides
- FNA—especially useful for masses

**Tx:** L-thyroxine (T4): 1.0–1.6 µg/kg/day; start slow and adjust dose based on TSH level

**Complications:** Myxedema coma, cretinism

## 7.16 KLINEFELTER'S SYNDROME

**Etiology:** Developmental abnormality causing hypogonadism, due to the presence of one or more supernumerary X chromosomes

**S/S:** Gynecomastia, sterility, lack of libido, ↓ body hair, excessive growth of long bones, +/− mental retardation, testes usually small and firm, penis and prostate are normal

**Dx:** Ejaculate contains no spermatozoa, urinary 17-ketosteroids ↓ → normal, serum testosterone ↓, LH and FSH ↑, estradiol ↑; chromosomal analysis needed to diagnose

**Tx:**
- Testosterone replacement for those whose secondary sexual characteristics have not developed
- Plastic surgery for gynecomastia if needed
- No treatment for sterility

**Complications:** None

## 7.17 OSTEOPOROSIS

**Etiology:** An absolute ↓ in the amount of bone present, due to an ↑ rate of bone resorption

**Risk Factors:** White race, females, early menopause, IBS, prolonged use of corticosteroids, phenytoin, renal failure, alcoholism, smoking, sedentary lifestyle, ↓ calcium/vitamin D, ↑ caffeine use

**S/S:** Asymptomatic until fractures occur

**Dx:**
- Bone-density scan—method of choice for diagnosis and to monitor response to treatment
- X-ray—significant mineral loss is present before osteopenia is noted on x-rays

**Tx:**
- Weight-bearing exercise, adequate dietary intake of calcium and vitamin D, HRT for postmenopausal women
- Lifestyle changes (stop tobacco use, ETOH use, ↓ caffeine use, evaluate for medications that ↑ risk)
- Medications—calcitonin, bisphosphonates

**Complications:** Fractures

## 7.18 PHEOCHROMOCYTOMA

**Etiology:** Adrenal tumor that produces, stores, and secretes catecholamines; malignant in 10% of cases

**S/S:** Hypertension, HA, sweating, palpitations, nervousness, tachycardia, fever, weight loss, hyperglycemia, orthostatic hypotension, hypotension/shock, arrhythmias, cardiomyopathy, heart failure, angina, MI

**Dx:**
- 24-hr urine—catecholamines, metanephrines; vanillylmandelic acid is generally diagnostic
- CT/MRI—to locate tumor
- ECG—nonspecific ST-T wave changes, prominent U waves, BBB, LV strain patterns

**Tx:**
- Resection is definitive cure; must use catecholamine-receptor blocking agent during surgery to prevent HTN crisis
- Medical management—nitroprusside, calcium channel blockers, ACE inhibitors
- Unresectable or malignant tumors—tyrosine hydroxylase (↓ catecholamine production)

**Complications:** Hypertensive crisis, severe drug reactions, recurrence (rare)

## 7.19 SYNDROME OF INAPPROPRIATE ANTIDIURETIC HORMONE (SIADH)

**Etiology:** Due to an interference in the osmotic suppression of ADH; leads to unchecked water reabsorption, which results in a low-volume, highly concentrated urine

**S/S:** Signs of hyponatremia (lethargy, anorexia, confusion, HA, N/V, focal neurologic deficits, convulsions, coma)

**Dx:**
- Labs—hyponatremia, serum osmolality < 275 mOsm/kg, urine osmolality > serum osmolality, urine sodium > 20 mmol/day, low uric acid
- Water-load test—determines if patient can excrete a water load by producing dilute urine; + if unable to excrete > 90% of 20 mL/kg water load in 4 hr and/or cannot dilute urine to < 100 mOsm/kg

**Tx:** Treat any underlying syndrome; fluid restriction (< 1000 mL/day); hypertonic saline (3%–5%) if severe hyponatremia (Na < 120 mmol/L); loop diuretics for severe ↓ urine output; demeclocycline (decreases water reabsorption)

**Complications:** Severe hyponatremia, death, central pontine demyelinosis (due to haphazard sodium infusion)

## 7.20 THYROID CARCINOMA

**Types:**
- Papillary (P)—75%; well differentiated, usually curable
- Follicular (F)—10%; common in iodine-deficient areas, functions like normal thyroid tissue, often curable
- Medullary (M)—10%; cancer of calcitonin-producing cells, associated with MEN II syndromes
- Anaplastic (A)—5%; poorly differentiated, aggressive, poor prognosis

**Etiology:** Associated with radiation to head and neck

**S/S:** Solitary nodule, +/– S/S of hyperthyroidism, rapid growth, history of head/neck radiation, nonmobile mass

**Dx:** Thyroid scan—"hot" usually benign, 10%–20% of "cold" are malignant; FNA is diagnostic

**Tx:**
- Surgical excision followed by radioactive iodine ablation of remaining thyroid tissue and potential metastases (except for anaplastic type), TSH suppression therapy for life
- M—advanced cases, radiation and chemotherapy for palliative treatment only
- A—radiation and radioactive iodine, but neither is very effective

**Complications:**
- P—slow-growing, generally only regional metastases, few recurrences after removal, most caught early with >90% survival
- F—> 50% have a 20-year survival
- M—< 50% have a 20-year survival
- A—early metastases, high mortality, with death within 6 months

## 7.21 THYROIDITIS

**Etiology:** Two groups:

1. Those due to specific cause (bacterial infection, tuberculosis, syphilis)
2. Those due to unknown cause (autoimmune or viral); de Quervain's; includes Hashimoto's (the most common type), postpartum, lymphocytic

**S/S:**

1. Infectious—severe pain, tenderness, redness, fluctuation over thyroid (rare type)
2. Nonspecific—acute, painful enlargement of the thyroid, +/– dysphagia, thyrotoxicosis and malaise; pain may radiate to ears, usually lasts for several weeks; Hashimoto's—painless insidious enlargement of thyroid, few pressure symptoms; thyroid is firm, symmetrically enlarged, lobulated, and nontender; usually normal thyroid function

**Dx:**

- Acute—↑ T4 & T3 resin uptake, leukocytosis, ↑ ESR, ↑ serum globulins
- Chronic—normal to low T4 & T3 resin uptake
- Radioiodine uptake—↓ subacute; ↑ chronic
- Thyroid autoantibodies—Hashimoto's

**Tx:** Antibiotics for suppurative; I&D if abscess is present; De Quervain's = ASA, +/– prednisone; Hashimoto's = levothyroxine, monitor for hypothyroid

**Complications:** Effects of mass on neck structures, hypothyroidism, carcinoma or lymphoma, Addison's disease, hypoparathyroidism, diabetes, pernicious anemia

## 7.22 TURNER'S SYNDROME

**Etiology:** Chromosomal disorder associated with absence of ovaries, due to a lack of one of the 2X chromosomes

**S/S:** Genital hypoplasia, primary amenorrhea, scant axillary and pubic hair, short stature, ↑ carrying angle, webbing of neck, "shield" chest with widely spaced nipples, cardiovascular disorders (coarctation of the aorta), osteoporosis, skeletal anomalies (short fourth metacarpals, exostosis of tibia), lymphedema of hands/feet

**Dx:** ↑ serum FSH and LH; chromosomal assay to confirm diagnosis

**Tx:**

- Estrogens +/– androgens may promote growth, but usually not significantly
- No treatment for sterility
- Treat associated anomalies as needed

**Complications:** Due to associated anomalies

# CHAPTER 8

# Neurologic System

## 8.1  ALZHEIMER'S DISEASE

**Etiology:** Progressive dementia of insidious onset characterized by atrophy of the cerebral cortex; genetic mutations have been implicated

**S/S:** Memory impairment; loss of reasoning abilities; difficulties with ADLs; decline in language function; decline in cognition; visuospatial disturbances; agitation

**Dx:**
- Definitive diagnosis can be made only on autopsy
- Probable diagnosis—inferred in patients who have progressive deterioration in cognitive ability without neurologic or medical cause
- Possible diagnosis—inferred in patients with progressive deterioration in cognitive ability but who have other medical problems present
- CT/MRI—atrophy of the cerebral cortex +/− vascular infarcts

**Tx:** Treatment is palliative; tacrine and donepezil may improve cognitive function; selegiline and α-tocopherol may delay progression

**Complications:** No true complications, only progression

## 8.2  AMYOTROPHIC LATERAL SCLEROSIS

**Etiology:** Degeneration of anterior horn motor neurons and corticospinal tracts, affects both upper and lower motor neurons

**S/S:**
- Weakness, cramping, aching; diffuse fasciculations, including tongue; gait problems; asymmetrical weakness/atrophy of hands; dysphagia, hoarseness; spares voluntary eye muscles and urinary sphincter
- Upper motor neuron signs—spasticity, hyperreflexia, upward Babinski reflex
- Lower motor neuron signs—flaccid paralysis, areflexia/hyporeflexia, fasciculations, downward Babinski

**Dx:**
- Clinical diagnosis
- EMG and nerve conduction studies
- CSF—+/− ↑ protein
- Muscle biopsy—shows denervation

**Tx:** Riluzole may prolong survival by 3–6 months; supportive care—monitor swallowing ability, tracheostomy to prevent aspiration, pulmonary toilet, G tube for feeding, PT, bracing, baclofen or diazepam for spasticity PRN

**Complications:** Pneumonia, DVT, PE, respiratory failure, death (median survival 3–4 years)

## 8.3 BELL'S PALSY

**Etiology:** Idiopathic facial paresis of lower motor neuron type; attributed to an inflammatory reaction involving the facial nerve

**S/S:** Characteristic facial paresis—comes on abruptly, may worsen over 1–2 days, pain about the ear, face feels stiff and pulled to one side, +/– ipsilateral restriction of eye closure and difficulty eating, ↓ fine facial movements, ↓ taste, +/– abnormally sensitive to sound

**Dx:** Clinical diagnosis

**Tx:**
- Most will recover without treatment; 60% will recover completely; only 10% will have permanent impairment
- Treatment consists of oral corticosteroids; should be started within 5 days of onset of symptoms

**Complications:** Incomplete resolution of symptoms

## 8.4 CEREBROVASCULAR ACCIDENT

**Etiology:**
- Ischemic strokes (> 80%)—thrombosis of an atherosclerotic vessel; embolism secondary to atrial fibrillation or paradoxical emboli; small vessel lacunar infarction
- Hemorrhagic strokes (15–20%)—intracerebral hemorrhage or subarachnoid hemorrhage

**S/S:**
- Acute onset of focal neurologic deficits; symptoms usually preceded by TRANSIENT ISCHEMIC ATTACK (TIA)
- Symptoms vary by area of circulation affected—carotid circulation (visual, language, motor or sensory disturbances); vertebrobasilar (visual, CN deficits, eye movement disturbances, impaired motor coordination, sensation, drop attacks, altered consciousness); +/– carotid bruit, heart murmur, irregular heartbeat

**Dx:**
- Emergent CT, infarcts—low-density (dark); blood more dense (white)
- Full workup to determine cause—ECG, echocardiogram, carotid US, labs (CBC, electrolytes, ESR, TFT, coagulation studies)

**Tx:**
- Thrombolytic therapy (rtPA)—must be given within 3 hr of onset of symptoms; hemorrhagic stroke must be ruled out prior to initiating therapy
- Avoid excess glucose
- BP management
- Emergency surgery (to release mass effect associated with swelling)
- Modify risk factors
- Hemorrhagic—mannitol, hyperventilation, head elevation

**Complications:** Severe neurologic disability, subsequent CVAs, death

## 8.5 CRANIAL NERVES

| CN # | Name | To Test |
|---|---|---|
| I | Olfactory | Smell |
| II | Optic | Visual acuity, visual fields, fundus |
| III | Oculomotor | EOM |
| IV | Trochlear | EOM |
| V | Trigeminal | Jaw strength |
| VI | Abducens | EOM |
| VII | Facial | Facial symmetry, nasolabial folds |
| VIII | Vestibulocochlear (Auditory) | Weber, Rinne, nystagmus |
| IX | Glossopharyngeal | Speech |
| X | Vagus | Soft palate elevation |
| XI | Spinal accessory | Shoulder shrug, head turning |
| XII | Hypoglossal | Tongue movement |

## 8.6 DEMENTIA AND DELIRIUM, COMPARISON

| Feature | Dementia | Delirium |
|---|---|---|
| Onset | Insidious | Rapid, often presents at night |
| Course | Stable deterioration | Fluctuates (↑ at night) |
| Sleep-wake cycle | Fragmented sleep | Disrupted (always) |
| Perception | Misperceptions absent | Misperceptions common (visual) |
| Awareness | Usually normal | Always impaired |
| Alertness | Usually normal | Fluctuates |

## 8.7 ENCEPHALITIS

**Etiology:** May be due to viral or bacterial infection of the brain; bacterial is usually due to partially treated bacterial meningitis

**S/S:** Fever, HA, N/V, malaise, stiff neck, ALOC, seizures, paresis, CN dysfunction

**Dx:** CSF—normal glucose, no bacteria; identification of virus in CSF is difficult but antibodies may be detected; in cases of multiple outbreaks, antibodies should be sought

**Tx:**
- Depends on exact cause, supportive for all patients
- HSV—acyclovir
- Syphilis—IV penicillin
- Toxoplasmosis—co-trimoxazole (Bactrim)

**Complications:** Permanent brain injury, death

## 8.8 GUILLAIN-BARRÉ SYNDROME

**Etiology:**
- Acquired inflammatory disorder of peripheral nerves; most cases are diseases of demyelination, frequently follows viral illness, *Campylobacter* infection, surgery, or immunizations
- Characterized by acute onset of progressive weakness in more than one limb; attacks may be mild (ataxia) or severe (rapid paralysis of bulbar and respiratory muscles)

**S/S:** Ataxia; progressive weakness of extremities (symmetrical, ascending, more severe proximally); hypoventilation due to weakness of respiratory muscles; ocular symptoms, swallowing difficulty; absence of DTRs; +/− severe, visceral pain

**Dx:**
- CSF—normal early, may show ↑ protein with few cells after 1 week
- EMG—diffuse demyelination and ↓ nerve conduction velocities

**Tx:** Emergent hospitalization; supportive treatment (intubation and mechanical ventilation PRN, PT); IVIG or plasmapheresis; may ↓ severity and duration

**Complications:** Residual weakness, recurrence, death

## 8.9 HEADACHE

**Types:** Three types of primary headaches:

- Migraine—common and classic (M)
- Tension (T)
- Cluster (C)

**Etiology:** Triggered by bright light, stress, diet, trauma, alcohol, OCP, exercise

**S/S:**

- Common M—throbbing pain, frontal or temporal, unilateral or bilateral; nausea; photophobia; no aura or neurologic deficits; may last for a day or longer
- Classic M—symptoms of common migraine + preceded by aura that lasts a few minutes, may include temporary neurologic deficits
- T—diffuse, bilateral pain; may last for hours to days
- C—severe unilateral pain, generally around eye, temple, or forehead; lasts minutes to hours; usually occurs at night; occurs daily for months, then remits for many months or years

**Dx:** Clinical diagnosis; in patient with no history of migraine and severe HA must rule out more sinister cause (infection, subarachnoid hemorrhage, tumor, subdural hematoma)

**Tx:**

- Identify triggers and modify reversible factors
- Acute attack—rest in dark quiet room, sumatriptan, ergotamines, NSAIDs, other analgesics, sedatives; antiemetics may be needed
- Prophylactic treatment—beta blockers, calcium channel blockers, tricyclic antidepressants, anticonvulsants

**Complications:** None

## 8.10 HUNTINGTON'S CHOREA

**Etiology:** Autosomal dominant mutation in chromosome 4; results in a loss of GABA neurons in the caudate and putamen; characterized by choreiform movements, mental status decline, personality changes

**S/S:**

- Involuntary choreic movements of hands and face—worse with voluntary movement, ↑ by emotional stimuli, disappears with sleep
- Dementia—memory loss, apathy
- Personality changes—agitation, psychosis, irritability, antisocial behavior
- Brisk reflexes
- Motor impersistence—inability to sustain motor act (tongue protrusion)

**Dx:**

- Clinical diagnosis
- CT/MRI—cerebral atrophy
- EEG—diffuse changes
- Diagnosis confirmed by genetic testing

**Tx:** No treatment available for this disease; neuroleptics, haloperidol, reserpine may be used to attempt to control choreic movements

**Complications:** Progressive course, eventually requires institutionalization

## 8.11 HYDROCEPHALUS, NORMAL PRESSURE

**Etiology:** Dilatation of the cerebral ventricles, usually secondary to some prior CNS insult (subarachnoid hemorrhage, head trauma, infection, tumors, aqueductal stenosis)

**S/S:**
- Classic triad—wobbly, wacky, wet; gait disturbance (apraxia), dementia, urinary incontinence
- Weakness, malaise, lethargy

**Dx:** Clinical diagnosis, confirmed by LP (normal or high-normal CSF pressure) and CT/MRI (enlarged ventricles and communicating hydrocephalus, narrowed cerebral sulci)

**Tx:** Removal of CSF via LP may provide temporary relief; ventriculoperitoneal shunt is definitive treatment

**Complications:** Infection, permanent brain damage

## 8.12 INTRACRANIAL HEMORRHAGE: EPIDURAL

**Etiology:** Usually due to trauma; bleeding site most commonly the middle meningeal artery, followed by the venous sinus

**S/S:** HA, ↓ LOC, ↓ motor coordination, pupillary changes; S/S usually develop within 24–96 hr of trauma

**Dx:** CT—will demonstrate hematoma between the dura and skull, usually will not cross suture line

**Tx:** Emergent evacuation of clot—usually accomplished via burr holes

**Complications:** Permanent brain injury, death, infection

## 8.13  INTRACRANIAL HEMORRHAGE: SUBDURAL

**Etiology:**
- Usually secondary to trauma, also may be due to minor trauma in a patient on anticoagulation therapy (commonly seen in elderly)
- May be acute or chronic (may occur up to 4 weeks after trauma)

**S/S:**
- Acute—ALOC, widening pulse pressure, dilated pupils, decorticate or decerebrate posturing
- Chronic—HA that worsens over time, ALOC, +/− hemiparesis, +/− pupillary dysfunction

**Dx:** CT—hematoma demonstrated between the dura and the brain matter; will usually extend beyond suture lines

**Tx:**
- Acute—emergent evacuation of hematoma via burr holes
- Chronic—evacuation may require craniotomy

**Complications:** Permanent brain injury, death, infection

## 8.14  INTRACRANIAL HEMORRHAGE: SUBARACHNOID

**Etiology:** Trauma is most common cause; also caused by ruptured intracerebral aneurysms, AVM, tumor, perimesencephalic hemorrhage and pituitary apoplexy

**S/S:**
- Classic presentation—sudden onset of worst HA in patient's life
- Nausea, photophobia, neck pain, altered mental status, syncope, coma, hypertension, ocular hemorrhage

**Dx:**
- CT of brain without contrast—acute blood will be bright white in subarachnoid space
- LP if CT is negative
- Cerebral angiogram is "gold standard"—demonstrates source of bleeding 85% of time
- Labs—coagulation studies, chemistries, blood type/screen

**Tx:** Stabilize patient; minimize external stimulation; control BP; treat hydrocephalus with ventriculostomy PRN; surgically secure any aneurysm; prevent vasospasm (nimodipine)

**Complications:** Rebleed of aneurysm (greater risk if not surgically secured); secondary vasospasm; severe brain injury with subsequent ↓ quality of life; death

## 8.15  MENINGITIS, BACTERIAL

**Etiology:** Serious infection of the CNS; can be caused by various organisms

**S/S:** Changes in mental status; fever; emesis; HA; tachycardia; hypotension; rash; stiff neck; KERNIG'S SIGN; BRUDZINSKI'S SIGN; focal neurologic deficits

**Dx:**
- Labs—leukocytosis
- CSF ↑ opening pressure, cloudy appearance, ↑ cell count, ↑ protein, ↓ glucose, +/− organisms on Gram's stain

**Tx:**
- Begin empiric treatment immediately, narrow antibiotic choice when cultures return
- 3rd-generation cephalosporin, +/− ampicillin; vancomycin if penicillin- or cephalosporin-resistant strains
- Treat dehydration aggressively, anticonvulsants as needed
- Prophylaxis for contacts of patients with meningococcal meningitis—rifampin

**Complications:** DIC, concurrent infections, hydrocephalus, deafness, seizures, blindness, cranial nerve palsies, death

## 8.16  MENINGOCOCCEMIA

**Etiology:** A fulminant form of septicemia without meningitis, caused by *Neisseria meningitides* groups A, B, C, Y, W-135

**S/S:** High fever, chills; HA; back, ABD, and extremity pain; N/V; +/− confusion, delirium; seizures; coma; shock

**Dx:**
- Lumbar puncture is diagnostic—cloudy to frankly purulent CSF with ↑ pressure and protein and ↓ glucose.
- Labs—PT and PTT; platelet count (for DIC)

**Tx:**
- IV antibiotics, aqueous penicillin G is 1st line, +/− 3rd-generation cephalosporin
- Antibiotics IV for 7–10 days or until patient has been afebrile for 5 days
- Treat complications as needed—IV fluid for hypovolemia, heparinization for DIC

**Complications:** DIC, cranial nerve damage, arthritis, hydrocephalus, myocarditis, nephritis

## 8.17 MENTAL STATUS CHANGES: GERIATRICS

**Normal Changes with Aging:** ↓ perception and impaired memory; ↓ coping capacity; impaired capacity for new learning; ↓ social and sexual interests; altered intellectual capacity

**Social Stressors:** Retirement, lowered socioeconomic status, constricted life space, constricted social contact and support, and constricted physical mobility

**Dementia:** Characterized by progressive impairment of memory, abstract thinking, problem solving, and deterioration of language and visual perceptual skills; most common cause is Alzheimer's (50%–60%)

**Delirium:** Cardinal feature is decreased attention and clouding of consciousness; most due to systemic conditions or toxic/metabolic derangements

**Workup:**
- Labs—CBC, chem profile, TFT, UA, ABG, ethanol level
- CXR, ECG, +/− EEG, CT scan or MRI of brain

**Tx:**
- Dementia—correct any potentially reversible processes; support group or psychotherapy if needed; treat medical problems judicially, avoid overmedicating
- Delirium—correct predisposing factors; DC any unnecessary medications, provide a safe environment, low-dose neuroleptics to assure patient safety when needed

## 8.18 MULTIPLE SCLEROSIS

**Etiology:**
- Acquired demyelinating disease of young adults; etiology unknown
- Destruction of myelin sheaths results in demyelination and inflammation of CNS white matter; multiple plaques of demyelination of different ages and in different locations are seen

**S/S:** Visual disturbances, weakness, sensory loss/paresthesias, vertigo, gait ataxia, spasticity, posterior column involvement, trigeminal neuralgia, euphoria/depression, incontinence/urinary retention, impotence, increased reflexes, Babinski reflex, LHERMITTE'S SIGN

**Dx:**
- MRI—multiple white matter abnormalities
- CSF—oligoclonal bands, ↑ IgG, normal to slightly ↑ protein
- Slowed evoked responses to visual, somatosensory, and other stimuli
- Diagnosis based on history + MRI and ancillary tests (CSF, visual evoked potentials)

**Tx:**
- Interferon-β and glatiramer—reduce relapse frequency and severity
- Corticosteroids—to treat relapses
- Symptomatic treatment—PT; prostheses/orthotics; amantadine (↓ fatigue); baclofen, tizanidine, clonidine, benzodiazepines (↓ spasticity); antidepressants; treat bladder dysfunction PRN; pain relief

**Complications:** Pneumonia, decubitus ulcers, permanent neurologic deficits

## 8.19 MYASTHENIA GRAVIS

**Etiology:** Autoimmune disease caused by development of antibodies to acetylcholine receptors on the postsynaptic neuromuscular junction; associated with thymic tumors, thyrotoxicosis, D-penicillamine usage, rheumatoid arthritis, SLE

**S/S:**
- Weakness—especially prominent following persistent activity; most often fluctuates but may be constant; respiratory muscle involvement results in hypoventilation and respiratory compromise; ocular muscles frequently involved, resulting in diplopia and ptosis; difficulty chewing and swallowing; limb weakness
- Fatigability—better in the morning, worse at end of day; improves with rest
- Normal reflexes and sensory function

**Dx:**
- Clinical diagnosis
- ANTICHOLINERGIC CHALLENGE confirms diagnosis
- EMG—repetitive nerve stimulation results in ↓ muscle responses
- CT of mediastinum—will show thymoma or thymic hyperplasia if present
- Labs—TSH

**Tx:**
- Anticholinesterases for symptomatic treatment
- Steroids, IVIG, immunosuppression and/or plasmapheresis
- Thymectomy may be curative (takes months to see effect)
- Avoid aminoglycosides, sedatives, beta blockers, and other meds that may ↑ weakness

**Complications:** Remissions and exacerbations of fluctuating weakness are common

## 8.20 PARALYSIS

**Definition:** Loss of muscle power, may be due to central disease, peripheral disease, disorders of neuromuscular transmission, or primary disorders of muscle

**Central Disease:**
- Upper motor neuron lesion—selective involvement of certain muscle groups, associated with spasticity, increased tendon reflexes, and extensor plantar responses
- Lower motor neuron lesion—leads to muscle wasting as well as weakness, flaccidity, and loss of tendon reflexes but no change in plantar responses (unless the neurons subserving them are directly involved); +/− fasciculations over affected muscles

**Peripheral Disease:** May involve the roots, plexus, or peripheral nerves; in distinguishing between a root, plexus, and peripheral nerve lesion, distribution of the motor deficit and any sensory changes are of particular importance

**Neuromuscular Transmission Disorders:** Weakness is patchy in distribution, often fluctuates over short periods of time, is not associated with sensory changes

**Myopathic Disorders:** Weakness is usually most marked proximally in the limbs, not associated with sensory loss or sphincter disturbance or accompanied by muscle wasting or loss of tendon reflexes

## 8.21 PARKINSON'S DISEASE

**Etiology:** Idiopathic paralysis agitans—a progressive, degenerative disease resulting from the loss of dopaminergic neurons in the substantia nigra and other CNS areas; characterized by slow movement, rigidity, and resting tremor

**S/S:**
- Classic triad—resting "pill-rolling" tremor, decreases with movement; cogwheel rigidity; bradykinesia
- Tremor, rigidity, flexed posture, loss of reflexes, bradykinesia, masked facies, unstable posture, difficulties with ADLs

**Dx:** Clinical diagnosis; clinical response to dopamine agonists suggests Parkinson's disease

**Tx:**
- Increasing levels of dopamine in the CNS—levodopa plus carbidopa
- Dopamine agonists and anticholinergics
- Bromocriptine, amantadine, selegiline, thalamotomy or deep brain stimulation

**Complications:** Medication side effects (dyskinesia), progressive disease with no cure

## 8.22 PERIPHERAL NEUROPATHIES

**Classification:** Based on the structure primarily affected; also may be due to disorders affecting the connective tissues of the nerves or the blood vessels supplying the nerves

**Predominant Pathologic Feature:** Axonal degeneration, paranodal, or segmental demyelination

**Mononeuropathies:**
- Due to injury or compression of nerves at a specific point along their course
- Sensory, motor, or mixed deficit, restricted to the portion of the nerve distal to the insult
- May be multiple mononeuropathies, which give a patchy multifocal presentation; due to vasculopathy (diabetes), infiltrative process (leprosy), radiation damage, or an immunologic disorder (brachial plexopathy)

**Polyneuropathies:** Lead to symmetrical sensory, motor, or mixed deficit that is worse distally; include hereditary, metabolic, and toxic disorders; best known is Guillain-Barré syndrome

**Inherited Neuropathies:** Charcot-Marie-Tooth disease, Friedreich's ataxia

**Neuropathies Associated with Systemic and Metabolic Disorders:** Diabetes, uremia, alcoholism, and nutritional deficiency

**Neuropathies Associated with Infectious and Inflammatory Diseases:** Leprosy, AIDS, sarcoidosis, polyarteritis, rheumatoid arthritis

**Neuropathies Associated with Malignant Diseases:** Guillain-Barré syndrome, chronic inflammatory polyneuropathy

**Mononeuropathies:** Carpal tunnel syndrome, tarsal tunnel syndrome, cubital tunnel syndrome

## 8.23  SEIZURE DISORDERS

**Types:**
- Grand mal—tonic-clonic, LOC, no aura
- Petit mal (absence)—brief loss of consciousness without loss of postural tone
- Jacksonian (partial)—focal motor symptoms begin in one hand or foot and "march up" the extremity

**Etiology:** Abnormal neuronal discharge leading to disturbance of cerebral function

**S/S:** Seizure activity +/− sensory or psychic aura; light-headedness; visual, olfactory, or gustatory changes; focal sensory disturbances; loss or impairment of consciousness; postictal state (confusion, agitation, prolonged alteration of consciousness); +/− urinary incontinence

**Dx:** EEG may be diagnostic, but negative study does not exclude seizure as a diagnosis; must rule out potential systemic causes of seizure (tumor, infection, drug overdose, or withdrawal)

**Tx:**
- Avoid alcohol and medications/drugs that may provoke seizure activity
- Anticonvulsant medication—valproate (grand mal and petit mal); phenytoin or Tegretol (jacksonian); ethosuximide (petit mal)

**Complications:** Status epilepticus, recurrence, trauma

## 8.24  STATUS EPILEPTICUS

**Etiology:** Single seizure lasting for more than 30 min or multiple seizures that occur without full recovery of consciousness between events

**S/S:** Convulsions most common, but other types of seizures are also possible

**Dx:**
- Labs—serum chemistries, drug levels, toxicology screen
- CT/MRI of brain
- LP—if imaging studies are negative
- Brain biopsy may be needed if lesion detected on scan

**Tx:**
- Eliminate seizure activity—IV phenytoin and/or benzodiazepines
- Thiamine—give first in alcoholics
- Glucose—if hypoglycemic
- Naloxone—if drug OD is possible
- Phenobarbital or high-dose benzodiazepines for persistent seizure activity
- Control airway—may require intubation if unable to stop seizure early

**Complications:** Permanent brain damage, cardiac arrhythmias, death

## 8.25 TEMPORAL ARTERITIS

**Etiology:** Inflammatory condition of unknown cause that affects all layers of extracranial artery walls

**S/S:** Unilateral temporal or diffuse HA; fever; malaise; arthralgias; weight loss; jaw/tongue claudications; sudden, temporary loss of vision; temporal or scalp pain/tenderness; indurated temporal artery; pale optic disk

**Dx:**
- Labs—+/− leukocytosis and/or anemia; ↑ ESR
- Biopsy of superficial temporal artery is diagnostic

**Tx:**
- High-dose corticosteroids
- Prednisone daily—titrate dose to keep ESR normal
- Methotrexate
- Maintain treatment for 1–2 years

**Complications:** Blindness

## 8.26 TRIGEMINAL NEURALGIA

**Etiology:** Idiopathic, on rare occasions may have a structural cause such as an anomalous artery or vein causing impingement on the nerve; other causes include MS or posterior fossa tumor

**S/S:**
- Episodes of sudden lancinating facial pain that arises near one side of the mouth and then shoots toward the ear, eye, or nostril on that side; pain may be triggered or precipitated by touch, movement, drafts, and eating
- Characterized by spontaneous remissions for several months or longer; however, as the disorder progresses, the episodes of pain are more frequent, with remissions shorter and less common; +/− dull ache may persist between episodes

**Dx:** Evoked potential testing and CSF analysis; CT or MRI of the brain only useful to rule out brain lesions

**Tx:** Carbamazepine is 1st line, phenytoin is 2nd line; may add baclofen to either if needed

**Complications:** Only complications are due to underlying cause if there is one; this is a progressive disease; persistent disabling pain may result later in its course

# CHAPTER 9

# Psychiatry and Behavioral Science

## 9.1 ADJUSTMENT DISORDER

**Definition:** A reaction to an identifiable psychosocial stressor or multiple stressors that occurs within 3 months of the onset of the stressors

**S/S:** Restlessness, irritability, fatigue, ↑ startle reaction, feelings of tension, inability to concentrate, sleep disturbances, somatic preoccupations

**Dx:** Considered a diagnosis of exclusion; 4 major decision-making processes are involved:

1. Establishing a relationship to a psychosocial stressor
2. Evaluating the level and duration of disturbance
3. Ruling out other mental disorders
4. Evaluating the context of the pt's total personality

**Tx:** Consists of 4 interventions:

1. Behavioral—stress reduction techniques, relaxation, or desensitization
2. Social—clarifying the problem (helps pt to see what needs to be done)
3. Psychological—supportive psychotherapy (emphasis on the here and now)
4. Medical—judicious use of sedatives for a limited time

**Prognosis:** Recurrent psychological disorders are 30%–60% more likely to develop in those who have had an episode of adjustment disorder

## 9.2 ALCOHOL WITHDRAWAL

**Etiology:** Sudden cessation of intake of alcohol after ingesting large amounts of alcohol for an extended time (7–8 pints of beer or 1 pint of spirits daily for several months)

**S/S:** Anxiety, ↓ cognition, tremulousness, irritability and hyperreactivity; DELIRIUM TREMENS, seizures

**Dx:** Clinical diagnosis based on physical exam findings and history of alcohol abuse

**Tx:**

- Pt should be hospitalized
- Adequate CNS depressants should be given to counteract the excitability
- Monitor VS and fluid and electrolytes
- +/− antipsychotic meds, seizure precautions, restraints PRN for pt safety
- Thiamine and folic acid supplementation should be given

**Complications:** Death due to aspiration, head injury 2° to seizure, cardiac events due to electrolyte imbalances

## 9.3 ALTERED MENTAL STATUS: GERIATRICS

**Etiology:** May be composed of any combination of disordered thinking, feeling, or behaving; may be on a functional or organic basis; an underlying organic factor is greater in an older population due to the higher prevalence of physical illness in this group than in the general population

**Differential Dx:**
- Cognitive dysfunction or pseudodementia—associated with underlying depression; may be differentiated from "true" dementia by the relative suddenness of onset, rapid progression, and responsiveness to antidepressant medications
- Paranoid delusions—tend to be mood-congruent in affective disorders and mood-incongruent in schizophrenia
- Medical illnesses—endocrinopathies, cancer, stroke, uremia, parkinsonism, pernicious anemia, CHF, and SLE may present as depression; manic symptoms may arise from brain tumors, MS, temporal lobe epilepsy
- Drugs—antihypertensives, benzodiazepines, antiparkinsonian agents, hormonal preparations, and anticancer agents may cause depression

**Dx:**
- Labs—TFTs, vitamin $B_{12}$ and folate levels, VDRL, ANA
- EEG, CT of head may be indicated

**Tx:**
- Depression—antidepressant medications, use 1/3 of normal dose, taper and DC after 6–9 months
- Arrange for therapy or support group, ECT as last resort
- Mania—neuroleptic meds or lithium as needed
- Anxiety—environmental manipulation, anxiolytics, sensitization if needed

## 9.4 BEREAVEMENT, ACUTE

**Five Stages of Bereavement:**
1. Alarm—a reflex physiologic alteration that occurs when acute stress exceeds the person's threshold of tolerance
2. Numbness—an adaptive defense mechanism that regulates the inflow of painful information so that it will not be overwhelming
3. Pining and searching—characterized by frequent hallucinations and pseudohallucinations of the deceased; stage accompanied by a high state of alertness and sensitivity to stimuli, restless movement, preoccupation with thoughts of the deceased, development of a perceptual set of the deceased, loss of interest in the outside world, calling for the person, and direction of attention to the environment where the person might be
4. Depression and disorganization—the loss becomes more real over time and despair sets in as searching for the lost person decreases
5. Recovery and reorganization—the final stage of grief, when the bereaved turns toward new goals and new relationships

**Mourning Lifeline:** Usually lasts from 6–18 months; at this point memories of the lost person become less painful and less intrusive

**Identification:** A normal process in which the bereaved adopts traits and mannerisms of the lost person in an attempt to be closer to him or her and keep memories alive

## 9.5 BIPOLAR DISORDER

**Etiology:** No clear etiology; it is postulated that changes in brain monoamine neurotransmitter metabolism and receptor function are involved

**S/S:**
- Past or present history of a manic episode characterized by a predominantly elevated, expansive, or irritable mood
- Manic episode—pt has abundant energy; engages in multiple activities and ventures at the same time; ventures appear genuinely creative, but as time goes on the pt loses the capacity to behave with reasonable caution and judgment; euphoria (sense of absolute conviction in a self-perceived talent or ability)

**Dx:** Clinical diagnosis, average age at onset 30 Y/O, with peak between 20 and 25, but may occur at any age between 6–65 years

**Tx:**
- Biomedical—lithium carbonate is the drug of choice for acute manic state, with therapeutic levels maintained between 0.5 and 1.0 mEq/L
- Psychosocial—therapy, must be gauged to the individual's needs based on other support (family, friends)

**Complications:** Suicide

## 9.6 COCAINE ABUSE

**Etiology:** Cocaine is a stimulant derived from the coca plant; preparations include powder for intranasal ingestion, "free base" or "crack" for smoking, and liquid for IV administration

**S/S:**
- Hyperactivity, sense of enhanced physical and mental capacity, sweating, tachycardia, ↑ BP, mydriasis, confusion and disorientation
- Chronic use—paranoid ideation with <u>DELUSIONS</u> <u>OF</u> <u>PARASITOSIS</u>, stereotypy, <u>BRUXISM</u>, psychoses (with aggressive responses); after stopping, pt may have paranoia and auditory hallucinations with small amounts of any stimulant (coffee, tea)

**Dx:**
- Clinical diagnosis, other organic causes for symptoms must be ruled out
- Labs—cocaine positive on drug screen

**Tx:**
- Medical—bromocriptine, carbamazepine, desipramine may help
- Psychological—treat psychosis, protect pt and others from danger if pt is violent
- Social—some type of structured program (e.g., Narcotics Anonymous)

**Complications:** Cardiovascular collapse, MI, TIA, CVA, seizures, hyperthermia, lung damage, obstetrical complications (spontaneous abortion, abruptio placentae, prematurity), teratogenic effects, delayed fetal growth, headaches, nasal septal erosions

## 9.7 DELUSIONAL (PARANOID) DISORDERS

**Etiology:** Idiopathic, possibly due to overwhelming stress in premorbid personality characterized by distrustfulness and hypersensitivity to slights

**S/S:** Insidious onset of delusional ideas (unrealistic fixed ideas that resist modification in the face of objective contradictory evidence or logic); pts function normally outside their circumscribed areas of abnormal thinking

**Dx:** Clinical diagnosis based on the following criteria:

1. Nonbizarre, superficially plausible delusions present for at least 1 month
2. Hallucinations, if present, are neither prominent nor persistent
3. There is an absence of strange or bizarre behavior
4. Schizophrenia, affective disorder, and organic disorders are ruled out

**Tx:** Antipsychotic medications (if pt will take them) should be tried; most important aspect is development of rapport and a trusting relationship between pt and provider

**Prognosis:** Poor; pts rarely give up their delusional beliefs; a satisfactory outcome is achieved if they can function in the community without feeling the need to act on or discuss their abnormal beliefs

## 9.8 DEPRESSION

**Etiology:**
- Depression is an ever-present reality of everyday life; it may be a final expression of genetic factors, developmental problems, or psychosocial stresses
- Pathologic depression occurs when the individual's coping ability is overwhelmed; then depression frequently expresses itself in some form of somatic complaint

**S/S:** Three major groups:

1. Reactive to psychosocial factors—a reaction to some exogenous adverse life situation (divorce, death of a loved one, loss of a job); anger produces a feeling of guilt; symptoms include sadness, anxiety, irritability, worry, lack of concentration, discouragement, and somatic complaints
2. Depressive disorders—includes the subsets of major depressive episodes (carbohydrate craving, hypersomnia) and dysthymia (persistent chronic depressive disturbance over a period of 2 yrs or more)
3. Bipolar disorders—episodes of mania and depression; these usually become manifest earlier than major depression (late teens or early adult life)

**Dx:** Clinical diagnosis

**Tx:** Includes medical (antidepressant medications, ECT), psychological (psychotherapy), social (flexible use of appropriate social services), and behavioral (desensitization, role-playing) support

**Complications:** Suicide

## 9.9 EATING DISORDERS: ANOREXIA NERVOSA

**Etiology:**
- Eating disorder characterized by weight 15% below expected, amenorrhea, and restriction of intake, binge eating, or purging behavior
- Restricting type—limits calorie intake
- Purging type—self-induced vomiting, laxative abuse, diuretic use

**S/S:** Weight loss; fatigue; amenorrhea; abdominal pain; intolerance of cold; hair loss; fainting spells; lanugo; bone pain; hypothermia

**Dx:**
- Excessive fear of gaining weight or being obese; distorted body image
- Interruption of menses for at least 3 consecutive months
- ECG—+/− bradycardia, prolonged QT interval, S/S of hypokalemia
- Labs—electrolyte abnormalities (varied)

**Tx:**
- Hospitalization indicated if weight is < 70%–75% of ideal, if pt has persistent suicidality, or with failure of outpatient treatment
- Weight restoration via a structured eating program
- Individual, group, or family therapy
- SSRIs may be helpful

**Complications:** > 10% mortality, depression, anxiety, obsessive-compulsive disorder, osteoporosis

## 9.10 EATING DISORDERS: BULIMIA NERVOSA

**Etiology:** Eating disorder characterized by recurrent episodes of binge eating, lack of control over eating, purging behaviors, and persistent overconcern with body shape, weight, fasting, and/or excessive exercise

**S/S:** Guilt about eating behaviors; abdominal pain and cramping; diarrhea (2° to laxative abuse); bloating; parotid gland enlargement; dental caries; calluses on knuckles; postural hypotension; muscle weakness and cramps (2° to hypokalemia)

**Dx:**
- Recurrent binge eating followed by inappropriate compensatory behaviors to prevent weight gain (purging, fasting, diuretic/laxative abuse, excess exercise) at least 2 times per week for at least 3 months
- ECG—+/− signs of hypokalemia
- Labs—electrolytes, CBC

**Tx:** Medical stabilization (correction of electrolytes and dehydration); educate pt and family; nutritional rehabilitation; cognitive behavioral therapy; +/− SSRIs

**Complications:** Relapse, dental caries, abdominal pain, electrolyte imbalances → arrhythmias → death

## 9.11 KÜBLER-ROSS STAGES OF IMPENDING DEATH

**Stage 1:** Denial and isolation—initial reaction is brief shock followed by a feeling that "it cannot be true"; serves to protect the pt from emotional overload

**Stage 2:** Anger—"why me?" anger is displaced and projected in all directions; family and friends receive hostility but should be aware that it is not meant for them

**Stage 3:** Bargaining—pt attempts to bargain for time or reduced pain, usually expressed as a pact with God or the fates; represents an extension of childhood attitude that being good may earn the pt special favors

**Stage 4:** Depression—both reactive (mourning for things already lost) and preparatory (mourning for the things left to lose—family and friends)

**Stage 5:** Acceptance—pt accepts the inevitability of death, begins to draw inward

**Note:** These are representative samples of the emotional reactions experienced by terminally ill pts, not inevitable occurrences

## 9.12 PANIC DISORDER

**Characteristics:** Short-lived, recurrent, unpredictable episodes of intense anxiety accompanied by marked physiologic manifestations

**Etiology:** Exact etiology unknown, possibly noradrenergic dysfunction plays a role in the pathogenesis

**S/S:** Unexpected episodes of intense anxiety along with physiologic signs (SOB, dizziness, palpitations/tachycardia, trembling, sweating, choking, nausea/ABD distress, flushes, chest pain or discomfort, fear of dying or going crazy, numbness or tingling sensations, derealization)

**Dx:**
- Must rule out medical problems that may produce anxiety—evaluate cardiovascular, respiratory, neurologic, hematologic, immunologic, and endocrine systems
- Discontinue any medications which may provoke anxiety—antispasmodics, cold medicines, thyroid supplements, digitalis, stimulants, antianxiety and antidepressant drugs
- Stop excessive use of caffeine, alcohol, and marijuana

**Tx:** Includes medical (antidepressant and antianxiety medications), behavioral (exposure therapy), and psychological (psychotherapy) treatments

**Complications:** Agoraphobia is often associated with untreated panic attacks

## 9.13 SCHIZOPHRENIA

**Etiology:**
- No single causative factor has been discovered
- Information from 3 main areas is important in the understanding of the pathogenesis of this disease: (1) genetics; (2) development of the individual before the illness; (3) biopsychosocial state of the person at the time of illness onset

**S/S:** Disorganization of a previous level of functioning; poor function in significant areas of routine daily living (work and social relations); lack of self-care; loss of grip on reality (leads to feelings of perplexity, isolation, anxiety, and terror); severe disturbances in language and communication, content of thought, perception, affect, sense of self, volition, relationship to the external world, and motor behavior

**Dx:** Clinical diagnosis based on the DSM-III-R diagnostic criteria

**Tx:**
- Combined drug and supportive therapy
- Medications—phenothiazines (1st line); other antipsychotics
- Supportive psychotherapy—family and individual therapy sessions with emphasis on developing a close and trusting relationship with the pt

**Complications:** Relapses

## 9.14 SCHIZOTYPAL PERSONALITY DISORDER

**Etiology:** Shares a genetic relationship with schizophrenia; entire etiology unclear

**S/S:** ↓ in ability to relate to others; peculiarities of ideation, appearance, and behavior; anxiety; depression; dysphoric moods; +/− reactive psychoses, eccentric convictions and magical thinking (superstition, clairvoyance, telepathy)

**Dx:** Clinical diagnosis

**Tx:** Antipsychotic medications and psychotherapy

**Complications:** Recurrence

## 9.15A SUICIDE

**Epidemiology:** Four major groups of people who attempt suicide:

1. Those who are overwhelmed by problems in their lives—they usually show great ambivalence; they do not really want to die but they don't want to continue to live as they are any longer
2. Those who are clearly attempting to control others—blatant attempt to hurt themselves in the presence of others, done to gain control over the other person
3. Those with severe depression—usually due to some life situation (illness, loss of a loved one or job), anxiety, panic, and fear are major findings; what looks like a dramatic improvement may be due to the pt's decision to commit suicide
4. Those with psychotic illness—these pts usually do not verbalize their concerns, they are unpredictable and are often successful in their suicidal attempts

**Gender:** Women attempt suicide twice as often as men, but men are up to 4 times more successful

**Clues to Suicide:**

- Verbal clues—direct (desire to die or "end it all"), or indirect statements ("You will be better off without me")
- Behavioral clues—ingesting small amounts of a potentially lethal drug or substance or putting one's affairs in order
- Situational clues—inherent in life experiences associated with major stress
- Syndromic clues—certain constellations of emotions that are commonly associated with suicide, acute delirium, psychotic disorders with impaired impulse control, in dependent people who view their suicide as a way to "really show them"

*(continued)*

## 9.15B SUICIDE, Continued

**Assessing Suicide Risk:**

- Ascertain the pt's characteristic mode of reacting to stress and whether he or she has ever considered or attempted suicide in response to a stressful event
- Evaluate presenting symptoms as possible somatic manifestations of depression
- If the pt has considered suicide in the past, explore frequency and extent of suicidal ideas; contemplated means of committing suicide; feelings associated with suicide and with the means of suicide; availability of means for committing suicide; relationship of suicidal ideation to ordinary acts of everyday life; pt's ability to imagine how loved ones would be affected by pt's death

**Assessing Degree of Suicide Risk:** To assess the severity of risk in a pt who has been labeled at risk:

- Transient thoughts about dying ("They'll miss me when I'm gone")—concern and caution are warranted, but pt is at low risk
- Sustained thoughts about dying and recurrent wishes for death (a painful habit that enables the person to deal with stress)—suicidal gestures are seen in this group, such as superficial wrist cutting or nonlethal OD
- Frustrated feelings and impulsive behavior (pt has little hope for support from his or her surroundings)—anger may be turned inward or outward
- Court of last resort (all emotional resources are depleted)—death is viewed as a way of avoiding further anguish
- The logical decision to die (sees suicide from a logical and philosophical point of view, "Death is inevitable, so why not now?")—this is the individual at highest risk

# CHAPTER 10

# Genitourinary System

## 10.1  ATHEROEMBOLIC RENAL DISEASE

**Etiology:** Atheromatous material obstructing the renal arteries

**Risk Factors:** Age > 60, atherosclerotic disease, arteriography

**S/S:** Renal failure of unknown etiology, HTN, <u>LIVEDO</u> <u>RETICULARIS</u>, painful muscle nodules, gangrene, +/− retinal emboli

**Dx:** Renal failure, confirmed only by biopsy

**Tx:** No treatment will reverse advanced renal failure; dialysis and/or transplant best treatments

**Complications:** Death

## 10.2  BLADDER CARCINOMA

**Etiology:**
- Transitional cell carcinoma is primary type, often of low-grade malignancy; metastases involve regional lymph nodes, bone, liver, and lungs
- 75% of bladder tumors occur in men > 50 Y/O, and usually arise at the base of the bladder and involve ureteral orifices and bladder neck

**S/S:** Hematuria, cystitis with frequency, urgency, and dysuria; suprapubic pain, obstruction of the ureters, hydronephrosis, +/− UTI and palpable tumor on bimanual examination

**Dx:**
- Anemia; urine—RBCs and WBCs; exfoliative cytology is confirmatory
- Cystograms usually show the tumor; cystoscopy and biopsy confirm the diagnosis
- US and CT are helpful in diagnosis and staging

**Tx:**
- Endoscopic transurethral resection of superficial and submucosal tumors is curative for many
- Cystectomy with ureterosigmoidostomy or another urinary diversion required for invasive tumors
- +/− radiation therapy for more anaplastic tumors
- Thiotepa, mitomycin, or doxorubicin instillation may eradicate superficial and papillary bladder epithelial tumors
- Metastatic disease—chemotherapy

**Complications:** Recurrence, ↑ malignancy

## 10.3 DIABETIC NEPHROPATHY

**Etiology:** Capillary basement membrane thickening of renal glomeruli → varying degrees of glomerulosclerosis and renal insufficiency

**S/S:** Proteinuria of varying severity → nephritic syndrome with edema and HTN → coronary and cerebral atherosclerosis

**Dx:** Labs—proteinuria, hypoalbuminemia, beta-lipoproteins; proteinuria does not diminish with progressive renal failure (10–11 g/day as creatinine clearance ↓)

**Tx:**
- Once HTN and proteinuria or early renal failure is present, glycemic control does not improve ultimate course of disease
- ACE inhibitors, restriction of dietary protein, dialysis (of limited value)
- Renal transplant is definitive treatment if no contraindications

**Complications:** Coronary and cerebral atherosclerosis, renal failure, death

## 10.4 EPIDIDYMITIS

**Etiology:** Inflammation of the epididymis, usually caused by sexually transmitted organisms (sexually active men < 35) or by common urinary pathogens (men > 35)

**S/S:** Diffuse groin or perineal pain; fever, chills, sweats; urethral discharge; dysuria, hematuria, frequency; very painful epididymis; PREHN'S SIGN

**Dx:**
- Clinical diagnosis
- Urethral Gram's stain, UA with C&S to determine pathogen
- CBC—leukocytosis

**Tx:**
- Adequate pain control (NSAIDs)
- Antibiotics—appropriate for cultures, or empirically (< 35 Tx for *Neisseria* and *Chlamydia;* > 35 cover urinary tract pathogens)
- Testicular support and elevation

**Complications:** Chronic pain, testicular infarction, abscess formation, infertility

## 10.5 GLOMERULONEPHRITIS

**Etiology:** Injury, inflammation, and necrosis of glomeruli resulting in abrupt onset of renal failure with rising serum creatinine, hypertension, hematuria, proteinuria due to IgA nephropathy, poststreptococcal glomerulonephritis, SLE, HCV, vasculitis, acute "allergic" interstitial nephritis

**S/S:** Hematuria, dark urine; proteinuria; mild to severe HTN; peripheral edema; oliguria or anuria; S/S of UREMIA; associated pulmonary hemorrhage in Goodpasture's disease, SLE, or vasculitis

**Dx:**
- Urinary sediment—RBCs, WBCs, casts, protein
- HTN, subacute or rapidly progressive renal failure
- Renal biopsy is diagnostic

**Tx:** Methylprednisolone; plasmapheresis, dialysis; diuretics; antihypertensives; treat underlying diseases

**Complications:** ESRD

## 10.6 HEMATURIA

**Etiology:** May be gross or microscopic; hematuria requires complete work-up

**S/S:** Dysuria (UTI, BPH, prostatitis, urethritis); flank pain (pyelonephritis, nephrolithiasis); fever (infections or malignancies); +/− menstrual irregularities; perineal and/or pelvic pain

**Dx:**
- UA—2–3 RBC PHPF is normal
- Urine C&S
- Creatinine, CBC, PT/PTT/INR
- Spiral CT, pelvic exam, renal US or IVP PRN

**Tx:** Depends on primary cause

**Complications:** None

## 10.7 INCONTINENCE

**Etiology:**
- Stress incontinence—inadequate bladder neck/sphincter tone
- Urge incontinence—due to spontaneous bladder contractions; may be central neurologic or local bladder disorder
- Overflow incontinence—overdistention of bladder due to outlet obstruction
- Detrusor muscle instability; UTI; medications

**S/S:** Inability to hold urine; urinary frequency or urgency; lack or awareness of impending incontinence; straining; irregular stream intensity or caliber; +/− dysuria or hematuria; may be associated with Valsalva or exercise; perineal/genital paresthesia suggests neurologic cause

**Dx:**
- UA—culture/sensitivity, cytology; postvoid residual
- Serum creatinine, glucose, calcium

- US—kidneys, bladder, pelvis
- Voiding cystourethrogram; urodynamic testing

**Tx:**
- Kegel exercises, physical therapy; timed voiding/volume restriction
- Treat UTI
- Neurologic/spinal cord dysfunction—catheterize regularly to prevent bladder distention if needed
- ↓ bladder contractility—improve detrusor muscle instability (Detrol, Ditropan, Tofranil)
- Surgical options if all else fails

**Complications:** UTI

## 10.8 NEPHROLITHIASIS

**Etiology:** Calcium oxalate stones (60%) secondary to increased concentration of stone-forming material in the urine

**S/S:** Severe, acute, colicky flank pain; hematuria; +/− pain radiating to testicle/labia; severe, acute urethral pain; N/V; CVA tenderness; fever/chills (if infection is present)

**Dx:**
- UA, urine pH, and urine cultures
- Spiral CT and abdominal x-ray—good for radiopaque stones
- US and IVP—for radiolucent stones

**Tx:**
- Hydration and analgesics if stone is passing
- Large stones—external shock-wave lithotripsy, cystoscopic or ureteroscopic laser lithotripsy, stenting, basket retrieval, or urolithotomy
- Treat infection if present
- Specific treatment for stone type: hypercalciuria = decrease sodium intake and thiazide diuretics; hyperoxaluria = decrease dietary oxalate; hyperuricosuria = alkalinize urine and allopurinol; cystinuria = penicillamine

**Complications:** Recurrence, infection, acute renal failure

## 10.9 NEPHROTIC SYNDROME

**Etiology:** Increased permeability of glomerulus leads to significant protein excretion due to primary renal disease, secondary to infection, renal manifestations of systemic disease

**S/S:** Peripheral and/or periorbital edema, hyperlipidemia with lipiduria, hypercoagulable state, infection (secondary to loss of IgG in urine)

**Dx:**
- Proteinuria, hypoalbuminemia, hyperlipidemia
- Urine sediment—casts, dysmorphic RBCs
- Serologic studies
- Renal biopsy—diagnostic

**Tx:**
- Fluid/electrolyte management
- +/− diuretics, statins, ACE inhibitors, or angiotension receptor blockers (may ↓ proteinuria and slow progression)
- Prednisone—14–16 week course minimum

**Complications:** Membranous nephropathy, DVT, thromboembolism, renal vein thrombosis, renal failure

## 10.10 PEYRONIE'S DISEASE

**Etiology:** Exact cause is unknown, dysplasia of the cavernous sheaths causing contractures of the penile sheath

**S/S:** Deviation of the erect penis to the involved side, +/− painful erections, difficult intromission

**Dx:** Clinical diagnosis

**Tx:**
- Surgical removal of the plaque and replacement with a patch graft may be successful or may worsen scarring
- Spontaneous resolution may occur, may take many months
- Local injections of high-potency corticosteroid may be effective
- Local ultrasonic treatment may relieve symptoms in some cases

**Complications:** Extension of fibrotic process into the corpus cavernosum, compromising tumescence distally

## 10.11 POLYCYSTIC KIDNEY DISEASE, ADULT

**Etiology:** Autosomal dominant mutations at PKD1 and PKD2; an autosomal recessive form caused by mutations on chromosome 6 causes in renal failure in childhood

**S/S:** Flank pain, gross hematuria, increased abdominal girth with palpable mass, +/− hypertension, +/− chronic renal failure, hepatic cysts, intracerebral or aortic aneurysms, diverticulosis, abdominal/inguinal hernias

**Dx:** Renal US/CT: enlarged kidneys with multiple cysts

**Tx:**
- Analgesia, bed rest (for hematuria), aggressive treatment for stones or infection, manage hypertension
- Kidney transplant is curative

**Complications:** Recurrent infections and stones, progressive renal failure leading to ESRD

## 10.12 RENAL CELL CARCINOMA

**Etiology:** Most arise from the proximal tubule epithelium; they account for > 90% of renal malignancies

**S/S:**
- Classic triad—hematuria, abdominal pain, abdominal or flank mass
- Fever, night sweats, weight loss, anemia, hypercalcemia, +/− signs of metastases

**Dx:**
- CT of abdomen and pelvis often diagnostic
- MRI useful to evaluate for metastases
- UA and urine cytology
- CXR and/or CT to evaluate for pulmonary metastases
- Bone scan to evaluate for bone metastases

**Tx:**
- Nephrectomy
- Interferon alpha, interleukin-2, and allogeneic stem cell transplants for refractory cases

**Staging:**
- Stage 1—confined within the renal capsule; 5-year survival, > 60%
- Stage 2—extends through capsule but only to Gerota's fascia; 5-year survival, > 60%
- Stage 3—renal vein, IVC, and/or local lymph node spread; 5-year survival, < 60%
- Stage 4—distant metastases, mean survival 1 year, 5-year survival, < 10%

**Complications:** Metastases, death

## 10.13  RENAL FAILURE: ACUTE

**Etiology:**
- Prerenal—renal hypoperfusion (dehydration, excessive diuresis, CHF, shock)
- Intrarenal—parenchymal disease (ATN, acute glomerulonephritis, atherosclerosis/thromboembolism, interstitial nephritis, medications)
- Postrenal obstruction—prostate enlargement, bladder or uretheral obstruction
- Vascular—renal artery stenosis, aortic dissection, renal venous thrombosis

**S/S:**
- Anuric, oliguric, or nonoliguric
- Lethargy; encephalopathy; HA; confusion; anorexia; N/V; fluid overload; edema; HF; hypertension; metabolic acidosis; hyperkalemia; arrhythmias; pericarditis; friction rub; asterixis; +/− fever

**Dx:**
- Elevated BUN and creatinine over hours to days
- UA—sediment gives clues to cause
- US/CT—evaluates for obstruction or hydronephrosis

**Tx:** Correct hydration, lytes, optimize hemodynamics; attempt diuresis with loop diuretics, +/− hemodiafiltration/dialysis

**Complications:** Multiorgan failure, ATN, ESRD

## 10.14  RENAL FAILURE: CHRONIC

**Etiology:** Gradual loss of renal function or sudden onset of rapidly progressive renal disease secondary to diabetic nephropathy, HTN, glomerulonephritis, renal cystic disease, congenital renal disease, myeloma, amyloidosis, atheroemboli, Fabry's disease, analgesic abuse

**S/S:**
- GFR 25–50: asymptomatic
- GFR 10–25: HTN, anemia, fluid retention, hyperkalemia, metabolic acidosis, hyperphosphatemia, hypocalcemia (leads to hyperparathyroidism with bone pain)
- GFR < 10: (ESRD) S/S of uremia

**Dx:**
- Serum creatinine: 0.8–1.2, normal (GFR > 90); 1.0–2.5, mild CKD (GFR 50–90); 1.2–4.0, moderate CKD (GFR 25–50); 2–8, severe CKD (GFR 10–25); 4–15, ESRD (GFR <10)
- Renal US, UA, renal biopsy (to determine etiology)

**Tx:**
- Control BP; treat specific disease; assess and treat reversible factors
- Fluid and sodium restriction, protein restriction, treat anemia, phosphate binders
- Dialysis and renal transplant for ESRD

**Complications:** Progression, cardiovascular disease, death

## 10.15  TUBULAR NECROSIS, ACUTE

**Etiology:**
- Injury or obstruction of the tubule of the nephron
- Ischemic injury (hemorrhage, shock, sepsis, prolonged dehydration, cardiopulmonary bypass) or nephrotoxins (aminoglycosides, contrast agents with iodine, NSAIDs, amphotericin B) are the most common causes

**S/S:** Decreased urine output, S/S of uremia, +/− fever

**Dx:** Oliguria, elevated BUN/creatinine; UA—coarse granular casts, renal epithelial cells

**Tx:** Hydration, hemodynamic support with pressors as needed; dialysis

**Complications:** Heart failure, multiorgan failure, sepsis, death

## 10.16  URINARY TRACT INFECTION

**Etiology:**
- Lower UTI—cystitis
- Upper UTI—pyelonephritis
- Common pathogens—*E. coli, Staphylococcus saprophyticus, Proteus, Klebsiella, Enterococcus* (community-acquired); *Pseudomonas, Klebsiella, E. coli, Proteus, Serratia, Candida* (catheter-associated)

**S/S:**
- Lower—frequency, urgency; dysuria; hematuria; N/V; abdominal pain; suprapubic tenderness; change in odor of urine; urinary retention
- Upper—all lower UTI signs **plus** fever/chills; flank pain; change in color of urine
- Urosepsis—hypotension, fever, mental status changes

**Dx:**
- UA—> 5–8 leukocytes, bacteriuria, ↑ leukocyte esterase, hematuria; +/− pyuria
- CBC—leukocytosis

**Tx:**
- Simple lower UTI—TMP-SMX or quinolone × 3 days; pregnancy—amoxicillin × 7 days
- Complicated UTI (severe illness or pyelonephritis)—IV ampicillin plus gentamicin or sulbactam; IV quinolone or 3rd generation cephalosporin
- Antipseudomonal if nosocomial infection
- Change catheter if catheter-associated infection
- Phenazopyridine—short-term urinary anesthesia to ↓ irritant symptoms

**Complications:** Urosepsis, death

# CHAPTER 11

# Dermatologic System

## 11.1  ACNE VULGARIS

**Etiology:** Disease of pilosebaceous follicles

**S/S:** Closed comedo (whitehead); open comedo (blackhead); inflammatory lesions; +/– pruritus

**Dx:** Clinical diagnosis

**Tx:**
- Topical retinoids, benzoyl peroxide, +/– antibiotics
- OCP for women
- Spironolactone
- Oral antibiotics for inflammatory acne—tetracycline; erythromycin; ampicillin most common
- Oral isotretinoin (Accutane)
- Surgical comedo extraction
- Dietary changes—avoid foods that exacerbate condition

**Complications:** Isotretinoin is teratogen; dry skin (complication of medications); cyst formation, pigmentary changes, scarring of skin

## 11.2  COLLAGEN VASCULAR DISORDERS

**Etiology:** A group of autoimmune disorders that have a genetic predisposition; all include widespread immunologic and inflammatory alterations of connective tissues

**S/S:** Synovitis, pleuritis, myocarditis, endocarditis, pericarditis, peritonitis, vasculitis, myositis, skin rash, alterations of connective tissues, nephritis

**Dx:** Labs: Coombs-positive hemolytic anemia, thrombocytopenia, leukopenia, immunoglobulin excesses or deficiencies, antinuclear antibodies, rheumatoid factors, cryoglobulins, false-positive serologic tests for syphilis, elevated muscle enzymes, alterations in serum complement

**Skin Involvement in Specific Diseases:**
- RA—palmar erythema, splinter hemorrhages under nails, subcutaneous nodules
- SLE—malar rash, discoid lupus, fingertip lesions, periungual erythema, nail fold infarcts, splinter hemorrhages, alopecia
- Scleroderma—diffuse fibrosis of the skin → skin is thickened and hidebound with loss of normal folds; telangiectasia, pigmentation and depigmentation are common
- Dermatomyositis—dusky red rash over the butterfly area of the face, neck, shoulders, upper chest and back, periorbital edema, purplish suffusion over the upper eyelids, subungual erythema, cuticular telangiectases, scaly patches over dorsal PIP and MCP joints

# 11.3 CUTANEOUS FUNGAL INFECTIONS

**Types:**
- Dermatophyte infections (*Tinea*)
- Yeast

**Etiology:**
- *Tinea*—infects hair, nails, stratum corneum
- Yeast infections—candidiasis (vaginal, oral, cutaneous) and pityriasis versicolor

**S/S:**
- *Tinea pedis:* pruritic, scaly, pink rash along sides of feet, soles, and between toes; *cruris:* pruritic, annular erythematous lesion on inner thigh and groin; *corporis:* affects torso, extremities, asymptomatic or pruritic, may present as papular, pustular, vesicular, scaly, or eczematous rash; *capitis:* asymptomatic patches of hair loss
- Pityriasis versicolor—asymptomatic maculopapular scales on upper trunk; precipitated by heat

**Dx:**
- *Tinea* infections—KOH prep: branching hyphae
- *Tinea capitis* may fluoresce green under Wood's lamp
- *Tinea versicolor*—KOH: short hyphae and round spores ("spaghetti and meatball" appearance); orange-gold fluorescence under Wood's lamp
- Candidiasis—KOH: yeast and pseudomycelia

**Tx:**
- *Tinea*—selenium sulfide shampoo; topical antifungals; low-potency steroid creams; systemic antifungals
- Pityriasis versicolor—selenium sulfide lotion; topical antifungals; oral ketoconazole
- Candidiasis—topical and oral antifungals

**Complications:** Systemic candidal infection—meningitis, endocarditis, lung infections

# 11.4 CUTANEOUS PARASITIC INFECTIONS

**Etiology:**
- Pediculosis (lice)—spread by physical contact or fomites
- Scabies—*Sarcoptes scabiei* mite, transmitted by personal contact or fomites; burrows into stratum corneum of skin and lays eggs

**S/S:**
- Pediculosis capitis—pruritus; eggs (nits) found on hair shafts; erythematous papules; excoriations; pediculosis corporis—pruritic, reddish, crusting papules; pediculosis pubis—may affect genital area, legs, buttocks, or face; blue macules with severe infection
- Scabies—reddish, crusting papules; present on genitals, buttocks, wrists/hands/fingers, axillae, or umbilicus; burrows appear as black dotted lines (2–15 mm long); intensely pruritic, especially at night

**Dx:**
- Pediculosis—identification of eggs on hair or body
- Scabies—microscopic identification of mites and ova within skin scrapings

**Tx:**
- Pediculosis—proper hygiene; clean linen and clothing; corticosteroid creams and antihistamines; permethrin or lindane shampoos; nit removal with fine-toothed comb
- Scabies—proper hygiene; clean linen and clothing; permethrin cream 5% from neck to toes; topical corticosteroids and antihistamines for pruritus

**Complications:** Secondary bacterial infection

## 11.5 DERMATITIS

**Etiology:**
- Allergic contact—type IV hypersensitivity reaction; non-allergic contact dermatitis may be caused by skin irritants
- Atopic—an allergic, pruritic dermatitis induced by specific triggers (type I hypersensitivity)
- Seborrheic—benign neoplasm of epidermis

**S/S:**
- Contact—initial erythema followed by intensely pruritic, papulovesicular rash; bullae, lymphadenopathy, fever; blistering, crusting, lichenification, scaling; location and shape of affected area suggest the specific allergen
- Atopic—intense pruritus with erythema, edematous papules, crusting, and excoriation; skin becomes chronically dry, hyperkeratotic, and lichenified; may result in exfoliation
- Seborrheic—asymptomatic unless irritated; slightly elevated colored lesions; range in color from white to yellow to red/brown/black; rough, greasy texture; mainly on scalp, face, and back

**Dx:** Patch testing; allergy testing in patients with food allergies or with severe reactions to airborne allergens; histologic examination if uncertainty exists

**Tx:**
- Avoid exposure; topical steroids or Burow's solution; antihistamines
- Severe disease—oral or IM steroids
- Atopic—steroids; Burow's solution; keep skin moisturized; oral antibiotics for secondary infection
- Seborrheic—treat only irritated lesions; cryotherapy with liquid nitrogen

**Complications:** Secondary bacterial infections

## 11.6 FOLLICULITIS

**Etiology:**
- Inflammation of hair follicles, usually due to *Staphylococcus aureus*
- Furuncle (boil)—when infection extends deep into follicle
- Carbuncles—infection of several connecting follicles with subcutaneous abscess formation

**S/S:**
- Light-colored pustules and papules with erythematous surroundings and a hair at the center; often pruritic and/or painful
- Furuncles—firm, tender, erythematous nodules 1–5 cm; become fluctuant; leave permanent scars
- Carbuncles—painful, may be > 10 cm; will drain from multiple follicular sites; lymphadenopathy, fever, malaise

**Dx:** Clinical diagnosis—culture to determine pathogen; biopsy for equivocal cases

**Tx:**
- Avoid friction and tight clothing; warm compresses
- Topical benzoyl peroxide, antibiotics, or steroid cream
- Oral antibiotics—cephalexin or erythromycin; ciprofloxacin (if *Pseudomonas*)
- Incision and drainage for furuncles

**Complications:** Spread, scarring, septic cavernous sinus thrombosis; secondary bacterial seeding—endocarditis, osteomyelitis, brain abscess, liver abscess

## 11.7 HIDRADENITIS SUPPURATIVA

**Etiology:** Inflammation of the apocrine sweat glands → obstruction and rupture of the ducts with painful local inflammation

**S/S:**
- Pain, fluctuance, sinus tract formation, purulent discharge
- Most common locations are axilla or groin, but may also be found around the nipples or anus

**Dx:** Clinical diagnosis

**Tx:**
- Avoid irritants (antiperspirants, deodorants)
- Rest, moist heat, oral antibiotics are key Tx in early course of disease
- Surgical excision (plastic surgery referral PRN)

**Complications:** Chronic infection with sinus tract formation

## 11.8 IMPETIGO: BULLOUS

**Etiology:** Staphylococci (Phage II)

**S/S:** Scattered, discrete thin-walled, easily ruptured vesicles and bullae, contain clear light to dark yellow fluid without surrounding erythema, located on the trunk

**Dx:** Gram's stain of early vesicle—Gram-positive cocci

**Tx:** Nafcillin, bacitracin, or mupirocin topically

**Complications:** None

## 11.9 IMPETIGO: VULGARIS

**Etiology:** Group A streptococci, *Staph. aureus,* or mixed infection

**S/S:** Transient thin-roofed vesicles → crusts, +/− erosions; golden-yellow color with "stuck on" crusts, scattered discrete lesions on face, arms, and legs, +/− regional lymphadenopathy

**Dx:**
- Clinical picture
- Labs—Gram-positive cocci on Gram's stain, group A streptococci, *Staph. aureus,* or mixed pathogens on culture

**Tx:** Penicillin is drug of choice, erythromycin for penicillin allergy

**Complications:** Glomerulonephritis

## 11.10 PSORIASIS

**Etiology:** Chronic disease of epidermal hyperproliferation resulting in immature cells

**S/S:** Silvery, scaly lesions; erythematous, sharply demarcated papules and plaques; symmetrical distribution; small to large, drop-like/guttate lesions; involves extensor surfaces; pruritus may or may not be present; pinpoint bleeding when scales are removed due to dilated dermal capillaries; nails pitted, separated from nail bed; +/− psoriatic arthritis

**Dx:**
- Skin biopsy is "gold standard" (if unable to diagnose by P/E)
- Psoriatic arthritis—x-rays: "pencil-in-cup" deformity of digits

**Tx:**
- Emollients and ointments; corticosteroid ointments or intralesion steroids during flare-ups
- Calcipotriol cream (vitamin D analog); anthralin or tar preparations
- Phototherapy—UVA; UVB, or PUVA
- Oral/IM methotrexate for severe disease; oral etretinate

**Complications:** None

## 11.11  SKIN CARCINOMA

**Etiology:**
- Malignant melanoma (MM)—neoplasm of melanocytes; superficial spreading (most common, occurs on back/legs); nodular sclerosing (rapid growth, often fatal); lentigo maligna (sun-exposed areas, common in elderly); acral lentigines (palms, soles, nail beds, occurs in blacks)
- Basal cell carcinoma (BCC)—malignancy of epidermal basal cells; slow growth, rare metastases but local ulceration
- Squamous cell carcinoma (SCC)—local invasion but rare metastases, may occur in burn scars

**S/S:**
- MM—solitary lesion, most frequently on back or other sun-exposed areas; flat or raised macule/nodule; satellite pigmentation and erythema; ulceration and bleeding
- BCC—papular or nodular lesion with central erosion, classic "rodent ulcer"; may have stippled ulceration, waxy pearly edges, and telangiectasias
- SCC—small, hard, reddened, conical nodule +/− ulceration; seen in areas of sun exposure; classically around the mouth/lips, face, and ears; rapidly growing lesion

**Dx:** Biopsy is diagnostic

**Tx:** Surgical excision with 1- to 2-cm margins; lymph node dissection if evidence of nodal disease; chemotherapy, interferon beta or interleukin-2 for metastases

**Complications:** Metastatic disease (melanoma)

## 11.12  STRAWBERRY NEVUS

**Etiology:** Proliferation of endothelial cells involving the dermis and/or subcutaneous tissues

**S/S:**
- 1.0- to 8.0-cm nodule, varies from bright red (superficial) to deep purple (deeper angioma)
- Soft to moderately firm lesion, may be localized or extend over the entire region
- Most common sites—face, trunk, legs, oral and vaginal mucous membranes

**Dx:** Clinical diagnosis

**Tx:**
- Most lesions appear within the first month of life, all within the first 9 months; lesions enlarge over the first year, then spontaneously disappear
- Mucous membrane lesions may not resolve and may require surgical excision
- Large lesions may benefit from cryosurgery, sclerosing solutions, or corticosteroids

**Complications:** Permanent disfigurement (more commonly due to overly aggressive surgical treatment); in very large deep lesions, especially on mucous membranes, may cause mass effect on surrounding structures

## 11.13 WARTS: COMMON

**Etiology:** Verruca vulgaris

**S/S:** Firm papules (1–10 mm average size), hyperkeratotic surface with vegetations, typically round isolated lesions, scattered lesions may appear on hands, fingers, knees; through hand lens, skin-colored lesions are noted to have "red dots"

**Dx:** Clinical diagnosis

**Tx:** Salicylic acid and lactic acid in collodion (small lesions); 40% salicylic acid plaster for 1 week (large lesions), liquid nitrogen, electrocautery, laser surgery

**Complications:** None

## 11.14 WARTS: FLAT

**Etiology:** Verruca plana, caused by HPV 1, 2, 3, 10, and 11

**S/S:** 1–5 mm papule, skin-colored to light brown; round, oval, polygonal, linear lesions noted at sites of minor trauma; always numerous discrete lesions to face, dorsum of hands, and shins

**Dx:** Clinical diagnosis

**Tx:** Lesions tend to disappear spontaneously; avoid aggressive destructive treatments; retinoic acid cream may be tried for long-standing or cosmetically unacceptable lesions

**Complications:** None

# CHAPTER 12

# Hematologic System

## 12.1 ANEMIA: APLASTIC

**Etiology:**
- A condition of bone marrow failure that arises from injury to or abnormal expression of the stem cell; leads to bone marrow becoming hypoplastic and development of pancytopenia
- Many causes—most common = autoimmune suppression of hematopoiesis by a T cell–mediated cellular mechanism
- Other causes—direct stem cell injury by radiation, chemotherapy, toxins, or drugs and SLE

**S/S:** Weakness, fatigue, vulnerability to bacterial infections, mucosal and skin bleeding, pallor, purpura, petechiae

**Dx:**
- Labs—pancytopenia, ↓ reticulocytes, RBC morphology is remarkable, neutrophils and platelets ↓
- Bone marrow aspirate and biopsy—hypocellular with scant amounts of normal hepatopoietic progenitors

**Tx:**
- Mild cases—RBC and platelet transfusions, antibiotics for infections
- Severe—adults < 30 Y/O, allogeneic bone marrow transplantation; adults > 40 Y/O or previous transfusions, antithymocyte globulin (ATG); ATG given IV in hospital over 5–8 days with transfusion and antibiotic support
- Androgens may be used, response is usually not as good as with other treatments

**Complications:** Death

## 12.2 ANEMIA: HEMOLYTIC

**Etiology:** Premature RBC destruction marked by excessive reticulocytosis

**S/S:**
- Fatigue, pallor, poor exercise tolerance; hemolytic symptoms (jaundice/icterus, hemoglobinuria, splenomegaly)
- Other symptoms depending on etiology: G6PD = hemolytic crises in response to oxidative stresses (fava beans, antimalarials, sulfonamides, vit K); hypersplenism = marked splenomegaly with stigmata of underlying disease; paroxysmal nocturnal hemoglobinuria = 10–15% have aplastic anemia, venous thromboses
- Symptoms of sickle cell anemia

**Dx:**
- Peripheral smear—abnormal RBC morphology
- Spherocytes—round RBCs without central pallor
- Target cells—↑ surface area:volume ratio (thalassemia, sickle cell disease)
- Acanthocytes—multiple spines on membrane (liver disease)
- Heinz bodies—precipitated hemoglobin in cytoplasm
- Sickle cells—sickle cell disease

**Tx:** Splenectomy—indications: hereditary spherocytosis, elliptocytosis, sickle cell disease, hypersplenism, TTP, steroid failure for immunologic hemolytic anemias; treat specific causes

**Complications:** Acute myelogenous leukemia

## 12.3  ANEMIA: IRON DEFICIENCY

**Etiology:** Poor iron intake, menstrual blood loss, states of rapid growth, blood donation, blood loss (GI bleed, Hodgkin's disease, excessive menstrual flow), pregnancy, malabsorption (gastrectomy, sprue, inflammatory bowel disease)

**S/S:**
- Fatigue, weakness, malaise; palpitations; pallor; ↓ exercise tolerance, SOB; pica
- Severe—mouth soreness (cheilosis), difficulty swallowing, spooning/curling of nails (koilonychias)
- May lead to high-output heart failure

**Dx:**
- Labs: ↓ serum iron (< 30 μg/dL), ↑ TIBC (> 360), ↓ ferritin (< 15), ↓ transferrin saturation (<1%)
- Peripheral smear—microcytic, hypochromic anemia; anisocytosis; poikilocytosis; +/− ↑ platelets
- Bone marrow—↓ sideroblasts

**Tx:**
- Treat underlying cause—iron supplements, stop blood loss, treat malabsorption
- Iron supplements, oral—ferrous sulfate 325 mg PO tid (between meals); parenteral—for severe iron deficiency if pt unable to tolerate high PO doses
- IM or IV iron dextran (must give test dose to check for allergic symptoms)

**Complications:** Heart failure

## 12.4  ANEMIA: MEGALOBLASTIC

**Etiology:** Deficiency of vitamin $B_{12}$ or folate, results in impaired DNA synthesis; vitamin $B_{12}$ deficiency usually due to poor dietary intake, ileal disease or resection, tropical sprue, fish tapeworm; folate deficiency most common in alcoholics or may be iatrogenic

**S/S:**
- Pallor, fatigue, weakness, ↓ exercise tolerance
- Vitamin $B_{12}$—thrombocytopenia (purpura); beefy red, smooth tongue; anorexia and weight loss; numbness, paresthesias, ataxia, sphincter disturbances, + Romberg and Babinski signs
- Folate—diarrhea, cheilosis, glossitis, signs of malnutrition

**Dx:**
- Labs—hemoglobin < 12 g/dL, MCV > 110
- Peripheral smear—anisocytosis, poikilocytosis, nucleated RBCs, hypersegmented WBCs, misshapen platelets
- Bone marrow—hypercellular marrow with ↓ myeloid-to-erythroid precursor ratio, ↓ megakaryocytes
- Vitamin $B_{12}$—< 100 pg/mL; folate < 4 ng/mL

**Tx:** Vitamin $B_{12}$ 1,000 μg/day IM for 7 days; folate 1 mg PO QD

**Complications:** Neurologic damage from $B_{12}$ deficiency

## 12.5 ANEMIA: PERNICIOUS

**Etiology:** Autoimmune destruction of parietal cells, leads to vitamin $B_{12}$ deficiency

**S/S:** Pallor, fatigue, weakness, ↓ exercise tolerance; thrombocytopenia (purpura); beefy red, smooth tongue; anorexia and weight loss; numbness, paresthesias, ataxia, sphincter disturbances, + Romberg and Babinski signs

**Dx:**
- Anti–parietal cell antibodies in 90% of cases; anti–intrinsic factor antibodies in 10%
- Schilling test—to distinguish nutritional or absorptive $B_{12}$ deficiency from pernicious anemia

**Tx:** IM vitamin $B_{12}$ supplementation and glucocorticoids

**Complications:** ↑ risk of gastric cancer

## 12.6 DISSEMINATED INTRAVASCULAR COAGULATION (DIC)

**Etiology:** Explosive, life-threatening bleeding disorder in which coagulation factors are haphazardly activated and degraded simultaneously, triggered by diffuse endothelial cell injury or release of tissue factors (amniotic fluid embolus, abruption, retained dead fetus, hemolysis, malignancy, trauma, infection/sepsis, acute pancreatitis, ARDS); involves both bleeding and thrombosis

**S/S:**
- Bleeding phenomena—skin/mucous membrane bleeding; hemorrhage from surgical scars, puncture sites, IV sites
- Thrombotic phenomena—gangrenous digits, genitalia, and nose; peripheral acrocyanosis

**Dx:**
- CBC—thrombocytopenia; fragmented RBCs
- ↑ PT/PTT; fibrin degradation products or fibrin split products
- ↑ D-dimer
- ↓ fibrinogen (with more bleeding)

**Tx:** Reverse underlying cause; control major symptoms: bleeding—FFP, platelets and/or heparin; thrombosis—IV heparin

**Complications:** Death

## 12.7 HEMOPHILIA

**Etiology:**
- Inherited disorder resulting in deficient or defective coagulation factors
- A—deficiency of coagulation factor VIII (most common type)
- B—(Christmas disease) deficiency of coagulation factor IX

**S/S:** Prolonged bleeding after surgery or trauma, hemarthrosis, oropharyngeal bleeding, CNS bleeds, hematuria

**Dx:**
- PTT—prolonged
- PT, platelet count, bleeding time—usually normal
- Assay of factor VIII or IX

**Tx:**
- Prevent trauma
- Avoid ASA and other antiplatelet drugs
- Treat bleeding episodes by supplementing coagulation factors: factor VIII or IX concentrates, FFP or cryoprecipitate, prothrombin protein complex (for hemophilia A only)

**Complications:** Transfusion-related infections, chronic liver disease

## 12.8 HODGKIN'S LYMPHOMA

**Etiology:** Malignancy of lymphoid tissue characterized by presence of Reed-Sternberg cells; EBV is suspected

**S/S:**
- Localized lymphadenopathy—central structures; firm, freely mobile, nontender; may be noted on CXR
- Constitutional symptoms—fever > 38° C (100.3°F); night sweats; weight loss (B symptoms)
- Nonspecific symptoms—rash, cough, CP, SOB, bone pain, GI discomfort, fatigue, malaise, pruritus

**Dx:** Lymph node biopsy is "gold standard"—RS cells (large cells with bilobed/multilobed nuclei and prominent nucleoli)

**Staging:**
- Stage I—1 lymphatic structure involved
- Stage II—> 1 lymphatic structure involved on same side of diaphragm
- Stage III—lymphatic involvement on both sides of diaphragm
- Stage IV—disseminated/marrow involvement
- B—presence of B symptoms (constitutional symptoms)
- E—extralymphatic spread

**Tx:** Stages I–II, radiation therapy; stages IIB–IV, chemotherapy

**Complications:** Myelodysplasia, AML

## 12.9 IDIOPATHIC THROMBOCYTOPENIC PURPURA (ITP)

**Etiology:** Autoimmune disorder in which IgG autoantibody is formed (in the spleen) that binds to platelets → destruction of platelets (occurs in the spleen)

**S/S:**
- Mucosal or skin bleeding, epistaxis, menorrhagia, purpura, petechiae
- Childhood onset may follow a viral infection, usually self-limited process
- Adult onset (20–50 Y/O) chronic disease, infrequently follows a viral disease

**Dx:**
- Labs—thrombocytopenia (platelet count < 10,000/μL)
- Peripheral smear—megathrombocytes
- Bone marrow aspirate—megakaryocytes

**Tx:** High-dose prednisone, which can be titrated as the platelet count increases, will not usually return to normal; splenectomy is definitive treatment; for patients who fail splenectomy, danazol may be used with fair results

**Complications:** Cerebral hemorrhage, life-threatening bleeding

## 12.10 LEUKEMIA, ACUTE

**Types:**
- Acute lymphoblastic leukemia (ALL)—lymphoid origin, classified L1–L3
- Acute myeloid leukemia (AML)—myeloid origin, classified M0–M7

**Etiology:** Malignancy of pluripotent hematopoietic stem cells of bone marrow; may be due to chromosome abnormalities, chromatin fragility, chemicals, x-ray treatment, drugs

**S/S:** Anemia (fatigue, pallor, palpitations); thrombocytopenia (epistaxis, bleeding, bruising); leukopenia (fever, infections); lymphadenopathy, hepatosplenomegaly; gingival hypertrophy/skin infiltration with leukemic cells (chloroma); bone pain; nonspecific symptoms (fatigue, fever, weakness, anorexia/weight loss)

**Dx:**
- CBC—WBC usually > 15,000; platelets usually < 100,000; normocytic normochromic anemia
- Bone marrow biopsy—> 30% blasts; ↑ nuclear:cytoplasmic ratio, prominent nucleoli, scant cytoplasm, hypogranulated
- LP in symptomatic AML and all ALL patients
- Blood type/HLA typing for possible treatment
- CXR, ECG, echo (evaluate LV ejection fraction)
- Labs—LFTs, RFTs, LDH, calcium, uric acid, lysozyme, phosphorus, PT/PTT

**Tx:** Chemotherapy, bone marrow transplant

**Complications:** DIC, death

## 12.11  LEUKEMIA, CHRONIC LYMPHOCYTIC

**Etiology:** A lymphoid malignancy of mature B cells

**S/S:** Lymphadenopathy, hepatosplenomegaly; frequent infections; anemia; thrombocytopenia; constitutional symptoms are uncommon

**Dx:**
- CBC—↑ WBCs with lymphocytosis (70%–90%)
- Bone marrow biopsy—> 30% lymphocytes; CD 19, 20, 5, or 23 on flow cytometry
- Associated with autoimmune hemolytic anemia and thrombocytopenia

**Tx:** Supportive care with IVIG and splenectomy; alkylating agents

**Staging:** Survival depends on staging:
- Stage 0—lymphocytosis only, 12-year survival
- Stage I—lymphocytosis and adenopathy, 9-year survival
- Stage II—lymphocytosis and splenomegaly, 7-year survival
- Stage III—anemia, 1- to 2-year survival
- Stage IV—thrombocytopenia, 1- to 2-year survival

## 12.12  MULTIPLE MYELOMA

**Etiology:** Malignancy of terminal differentiated B cells or plasma cells, related to radiation exposure and/or chronic antigenic stimulation

**S/S:** Bone pain; recurrent pneumonia and pyelonephritis; anemia; neurologic symptoms (hypercalcemia, hyperviscosity, peripheral nerve infiltration)

**Dx:**
- Classic triad—marrow plasmacytosis; lytic bone lesions; serum or urine M protein spike on protein electrophoresis in gamma region
- CBC; bone marrow biopsy/aspirate; serum and urine protein electrophoresis; quantitative immunoglobulins; labs (RFTs, chemistries, calcium, uric acid, alkaline phosphatase, $\beta_2$ microglobulin, LDH)
- Urine tests (24-hr urine for protein, Bence-Jones protein);
- CXR and bone x-rays

**Tx:**
- Localized plasmacytomas and pathologic fractures/cord compression treated with radiation therapy
- Myeloma treatment—chemotherapy; bisphosphonates (for bony lesions); renal protective measures (fluids, allopurinol, avoid IV dye); plasmapheresis for hyperviscosity; bone marrow transplant for chemoresponsive disease

**Staging:**
- Stage I (mean survival, 5 years)—Hb > 10 g/dL; serum Ca < 12 mg/dL; normal bone x-ray or solitary lesion; low M component (in urine/blood)
- Stage II (mean survival, 4.5 years)—patients not fitting into stages I or III
- Stage III (mean survival, 1–2 years)—Hb < 8.5 g/dL; serum Ca > 12 mg/dL; advanced lytic bone lesions; high M component

## 12.13  NON-HODGKIN'S LYMPHOMA

**Etiology:** Malignancy of lymphoid cells that reside in lymphoid tissues, 90% are of B-cell origin

**S/S:**
- Localized, persistent lymphadenopathy—painless, > 1 cm for 4 weeks, peripheral (axillary, epitrochlear, abdominal), non-contiguous spread
- Constitutional symptoms—fever, night sweats, weight loss >10% in 6 months (B symptoms)
- Nonspecific symptoms—fatigue, malaise, pruritus
- Symptoms of localized compression—cough, chest discomfort, GI discomfort

**Dx:** Lymph node biopsy is diagnostic; flow cytometry (CD15+ and CD30+ on Reed-Sternberg cell)

**Tx:**
- Treatment is determined by histology
- Aggressive—combination chemotherapy
- Indolent—observation only if patient is asymptomatic
- Salvage treatment—allograft bone marrow transplant

**Complications:** Death

## 12.14  POLYCYTHEMIA VERA

**Etiology:** Acquired myeloproliferative disorder, causes overproduction of all 3 hematopoietic cell lines

**S/S:** Headache, dizziness, tinnitus, blurred vision, fatigue, generalized pruritus, epistaxis, plethora and engorged retinal veins, splenomegaly

**Dx:**
- Labs—hematocrit > 60%, WBC ↑, platelet count ↑, RBC mass ↑, ↑ $B_{12}$ levels, ↑ uric acid
- Bone marrow aspirate—hypercellular with panhyperplasia of all hematopoietic elements, iron stores absent, ↑ megakaryocytes

**Tx:** Phlebotomy—1 unit of blood removed weekly until hematocrit is < 45%, then as needed to maintain; myelosuppressive therapy may be used if high phlebotomy requirement or marked thrombocytosis and intractable pruritus

**Complications:** Thrombosis, increased bleeding, peptic ulcer disease, GI bleeding, hyperuricemia, gout

## 12.15 SICKLE CELL DISEASE

**Etiology:** Inherited disorder resulting in production of defective hemoglobin, which leads to occlusions and infarcts of the spleen, brain, kidney, lung, and other organs

**S/S:**
- Pallor, fatigue, ↓ exercise tolerance; rheologic manifestations (<u>DACTYLITIS</u>, leg ulcers, priapism, pulmonary, cerebral, and splenic emboli, retinal vessel obstruction, blindness, aseptic necrosis); hemolysis (jaundice, gallstones, cholecystitis)
- Crisis—skeletal pain, fever, massive pooling of RBCs (acute fall in hemoglobin), jaundice

**Dx:** Peripheral smear—microcytic, hypochromic anemia, sickled cells; ↑ reticulocyte count; hemoglobin electrophoresis is diagnostic

**Tx:**
- Symptomatic support—avoid triggers (infection, fever, hypoxia, dehydration, high altitude); folic acid supplementation; *Haemophilus influenzae* and *Pneumococcus* vaccines; PCN prophylaxis to prevent pneumococcal sepsis (until age 6)
- Leg ulcers/painful crises—bed rest, skin grafts, hydration, analgesics
- Transfusions as needed
- Antisickling agents—hydroxyurea
- Allogeneic bone marrow transplant; broad-spectrum antibiotics in infections

**Complications:** Painful crisis, sequestration crisis (acute fall in hemoglobin), acute chest syndrome (fever, chest pain, dyspnea, pulmonary infiltration), death

## 12.16 THALASSEMIA

**Types:**
- Alpha thalassemia
- Beta thalassemia

**Etiology:** Genetic disorder resulting in ↓ amounts of functional hemoglobin

**S/S:**
- Pallor, fatigue, ↓ exercise tolerance
- Alpha—deletion of all 4 alpha genes = in utero death from hydrops fetalis; deletion of 3 alpha genes = severe anemia with signs of hemolysis; deletion of 2 alpha genes = mild anemia; deletion of 1 alpha gene = silent carrier
- Beta—major: severe anemia and bone changes; chipmunk face (frontal bossing), copper-colored skin; minor: microcytic anemia

**Dx:** Peripheral smear—anemia; microcytosis; hypochromia; abnormal cells; hemoglobin electrophoresis is diagnostic

**Tx:**
- Supportive therapy for anemia, genetic counseling, antenatal testing
- Transfusions as needed
- Splenectomy—for ↑ need for transfusions or clinical signs of hemolysis
- Beta thalassemia—folic acid supplementation, bone marrow transplant

**Complications:** Severe hemolysis, hydrops fetalis, death

## 12.17 THROMBOCYTOPENIA

**Etiology:**
- Decreased platelet count due to ↓ marrow production, ↑ splenic sequestration, or accelerated destruction of platelets
- Immune platelet destruction—ITP, infection, drugs
- Nonimmune platelet destruction—vasculitis, DIC, TTP, HUS, intravascular prostheses

**S/S:** Superficial bleeding (easy bruising, petechiae, epistaxis, menorrhagia), splenomegaly (if splenic sequestration)

**Dx:**
- CBC—↓ platelet count
- Bone marrow—↓ megakaryocytes
- History of viral illness (for ITP)
- PT/PTT, fibrinogen, D-dimer

**Tx:**
- TTP—HUS—plasmapheresis
- ITP—steroids, IVIG and/or antiRhD; splenectomy; cytotoxic drugs (controversial)
- DIC—treat underlying cause
- Stop any offending drug
- Platelet count < 20,000/µL, transfuse platelets; < 50,000/µL plus active bleeding, transfuse

**Complications:** Recurrence, hypovolemic shock

## 12.18 VON WILLEBRAND'S DISEASE

**Types:**
- Type I—autosomal dominant, deficiency of VWF
- Type II—autosomal dominant, defective VWF
- Type III—autosomal recessive, complete absence of VWF

**Etiology:** Absence of VWF results in failure to form a primary platelet plug

**S/S:** Prolonged bleeding, superficial bleeding due to failure to form platelet plug (petechiae, purpura, easy bruising, oropharyngeal bleeding, epistaxis, GI bleeding, menorrhagia)

**Dx:**
- Bleeding time—prolonged
- VWF assay—VWF antigen immunoassay; VWF ristocetin cofactor assay; factor VIII assay
- Electron microscopic assessment of platelet granules

**Tx:** Administer factor VIII concentrates; desmopressin acetate (DDAVP, synthetic analog of ADH, induces release of VWF); dialysis for uremia; if drug-induced, stop offending drug

**Complications:** Hypovolemic shock, iron deficiency (if excessive blood loss)

# CHAPTER 13

# Infectious Disease

## 13.1 ANTHRAX

**Types:**
- Cutaneous (C)
- Pulmonary (P)
- GI (G)

**Etiology:** *Bacillus anthracis* (GPR)

**S/S:**
- C—painless reddish papule that becomes surrounded by erythema and vesicles, +/− systemic symptoms
- P—fever, chills, fatigue, HA, cough, myalgias, dyspnea (sudden onset), cyanosis, mental status changes, coma, death
- G—oropharyngeal infection (sore throat, dysphagia, fever, lymphadenopathy), intestinal infection (N/V, fever, abdominal pain, hematemesis, bloody diarrhea, ascites)

**Dx:**
- Definitive diagnosis by isolation of bacteria from vesicles, sputum, vomitus, feces, or ascitic fluid
- CXR may show widened mediastinum and diffuse patchy infiltrates (P)
- Blood cultures may be positive in all types

**Tx:**
- PCN is antibiotic of choice—C—oral for mild cases, IV for severe; P and G need IV
- Alternative medications—ciprofloxacin, tetracycline, erythromycin, chloramphenicol

**Complications:** Sepsis, shock, meningitis, death

## 13.2 CELLULITIS

**Etiology:** Infection of skin and soft tissue, causes local cytokine release, which mediates local and systemic signs and symptoms; common pathogens: *Strep., Staph., Haemophilus influenzae* (in children)

**S/S:** Redness and warmth of skin and soft tissues, tender lymphadenopathy, lymphangitis, +/− abscess, fever, rigors, +/− mental status changes (in elderly)

**Dx:**
- Clinical diagnosis
- With systemic symptoms, obtain blood cultures
- Suspected osteomyelitis = local x-ray, bone scan or MRI
- Periorbital/orbital involvement = head CT

**Tx:**
- Antibiotics—cover *Strep.* and *Staph.* for 7–14 days
- Adjust antibiotics as needed if no response within first 48–72 hr
- Diabetics—ampicillin/sulbactam (Unasyn), strict glucose control

**Complications:** Local abscess formation, osteomyelitis, lymphatic obstruction, periorbital/orbital infection, cavernous sinus thrombosis, brain abscess

## 13.3  CROUP (LARYNGOTRACHEOBRONCHITIS)

**Etiology:** Viral infection (usually parainfluenza virus) of the subglottal area

**S/S:** "Seal bark" cough, inspiratory and expiratory stridor, xiphoid and suprasternal retraction

**Dx:**
- Clinical diagnosis
- CXR—"pencil sign" (narrowed subglottic airway)
- Labs–leukocytosis, initially → leukopenia and lymphocytosis

**Tx:** Cool humidified oxygen, hydration, dexamethasone, ventilatory assistance PRN

**Complications:** Complete airway obstruction, death

## 13.4  HUMAN IMMUNODEFICIENCY VIRUS (HIV)

**Etiology:** Retrovirus that infects CD4 T-helper cells, resulting in humoral and cellular immune deficiency and the development of multiple opportunistic and nonopportunistic infections; transmitted by blood products, sexual contact, IV drug use, perinatal infection, breast-feeding, and open wound–fluid interchange

**S/S:**
- Initial presentation is flu-like syndrome that occurs within 12 weeks of infection (fever, chills, cough, myalgias, adenopathy)
- Asymptomatic period of 2–10+ years
- Opportunistic infections usually begin to occur once CD4 cell count drops—URIs, UTIs, diarrhea, TB, meningitis, skin infections, abscesses, lymphoma, squamous cell cancer, Kaposi's sarcoma, new-onset thrombocytopenia, Bell's palsy

**Dx:** Positive ELISA and Western blot tests are diagnostic; viral load and CD4 counts every 3–6 months to follow progression of disease

**Tx:**
- Antiretrovirals—AZT, ddI, d4T, 3TC, efavirenz, indinavir
- Begin treatment of asymptomatic pts when CD4 < 350 or viral load > 30,000
- Triple therapy is rule to follow to avoid/prolong onset of resistance

**Complications:** Progressive multifocal leukoencephalopathy, malignancies, psychosis, HIV dementia, wasting syndrome, depression, severe anemia, ITP, death

## 13.5A IMMUNIZATION SCHEDULE: ADULTS

**Types:**
- Influenza—administered yearly, recommended for those > 50, health care workers, nursing home residents, high-risk persons' housemates
- *Pneumococcus*—one dose for immunocompetent persons > 65; revaccinate after age 65 if pt has cardiac, pulmonary, or liver disease, diabetes, CSF leak; also immunocompromised and long-term care pts
- Tetanus-diphtheria—recommended every 10 years for all
- Hepatitis B—3-dose vaccine, recommended for at-risk persons (health care workers, IVDA pts, multiple sexual partners, travelers, immunocompromised, dialysis pts)
- Hepatitis A—2-dose vaccine, recommended for travelers, day-care workers, pts with chronic liver disease, food handlers
- MMR—2-dose vaccine, recommended for fertile women, college students, health care workers, international travelers; 1-dose vaccine for other adults born after 1957
- Varicella—2-dose vaccine for those without documented immunity or at high risk (health care workers, fertile women, travelers, teachers, military, those in correctional facilities)

**Side Effects:**
- Local tenderness at administration site, low-grade fever, malaise; rare association with Guillain-Barré syndrome (influenza)
- Those with anaphylaxis to eggs or neomycin should avoid MMR
- True contraindications are rare, include severe hypersensitivity reactions (anaphylaxis, neurologic sequelae)

*(continued)*

## 13.5B IMMUNIZATION SCHEDULE: ADULTS, Continued

**Alternative Tx:**
- Influenza—amantadine 200 mg qd until 24–48 hr after symptoms resolve; *Pneumococcus,* fluoroquinolones, cephalosporin for 14 days
- Td—after exposure to tetanus = clean wounds + Td and TIG; after exposure to diphtheria = antitoxin, 14-day course of PCN
- Hepatitis B—HBIG and vaccine series following exposure; for disease, 1-year course of lamivudine or 6–24 months of interferon alpha
- Hepatitis A—hepatitis A gamma globulin for 1 dose (protective if within 2 weeks of exposure)
- MMR—after exposure to measles, immunoglobulin followed 6 months later by MMR
- Varicella—after exposure, consider vaccine; after exposure for pregnant or immunocompromised pts, VZIG, acyclovir, famciclovir, or valacyclovir for severe cases

**Efficacy:**
- Influenza—estimated at > 95% for elderly
- *Pneumococcus*—estimated at 70% in elderly (wanes after 5 years, but role of booster unclear)

**Complications:**
- Avoid MMR or varicella vaccine for at least 5 months after administration of immune globulin; if MMR or varicella vaccine given first, hold immune globulin for at least 2 weeks
- Immunizations in pregnancy—avoid live virus vaccines during pregnancy, although with MMR and varicella there have been no documented cases from inadvertent vaccination in pregnancy

## 13.6 IMMUNIZATION SCHEDULE: PEDIATRICS

**Routine Schedule:**

| | | | | | | | |
|---|---|---|---|---|---|---|---|
| Birth | HBV (1) | | | | | | |
| 2 Mo | HBV (2) | DTaP (1) | Hib (1) | IPV (1) | PCV (1) | | |
| 4 Mo | | DTaP (2) | Hib (2) | IPV (2) | PCV (2) | | |
| 6 Mo | | DTaP (3) | Hib (3) | | PCV (3) | | |
| 6–18 Mo | HBV (3) | | | IPV (3) | | | |
| 12–15 Mo | | | Hib (4) | | PCV (4) | MMR (1) | |
| > 12 Mo | | | | | | | Varicella |
| 15–18 Mo | | DTaP (4) | | | | | |
| 4–6 Yrs | | DTaP (5) | | IPV (4) | | MMR (2) | |
| Q 10 Yrs | | | | | | | Td |

Key:
HBV — Hepatitis B virus
DTaP — Diphtheria, tetanus, and acellular pertussis
Hib — *Haemophilus influenzae* type B
IPV — Inactivated polio virus
PCV — Conjugated seven-valent pneumococcal
MMR — Measles, mumps, rubella
Td — Tetanus toxoid

## 13.7 INFLUENZA

**Etiology:** Acute respiratory illness caused by influenza viruses

**S/S:** High fever, general malaise, myalgias, severe frontal HA, cough, chest congestion, sore throat, photophobia, pain with eye motion, cervical lymphadenopathy, +/− myocarditis or encephalitis/meningitis, bacterial superinfection (SOB, chest tightness, prostration)

**Dx:**
- Rapid influenza test—50%–80% sensitivity
- CXR—diffuse atypical infiltrates
- Labs—leukopenia or lymphocytosis

**Tx:**
- Symptomatic treatment
- Avoid ASA in children, can result in Reye's syndrome
- Goal of Tx—keep ideal oxygenation and prevent bacterial superinfection
- Antiviral medications may ↓ severity and length of infection

**Complications:** Bacterial superinfection → death

## 13.8 LYME DISEASE

**Etiology:** *Borrelia burgdorferi,* transmitted by ticks

**S/S:**
- Stage I—ERYTHEMA MIGRANS
- Stage II—2–4 weeks after stage I, hematogenous spread, HA, fatigue, sore throat, fever/chills, muscle aches, hepatitis, meningitis, Bell's palsy, polyneuropathy, carditis, AV block
- Stage III—months to years later, frank arthritis, encephalopathy (loss of memory, mood changes, sleep changes), ACRODERMATITIS CHRONICA ATROPHICANS

**Dx:**
- Stage I—clinical diagnosis
- Stage II—LP, lymphocytic pleocytosis; CSF exam for IgM and IgG; ECG, +/− AV block
- Stage III—serologies

**Tx:**
- Stage I—doxycycline for 21 days PO
- Stages II & III—IV or PO antibiotics; if arrhythmias, IV antibiotics; +/− pacemaker PRN

**Complications:** Arthritis, AV blocks, arrhythmias

## 13.9 MONONUCLEOSIS, INFECTIOUS

**Etiology:** Acute infection due to Epstein-Barr virus (a herpesvirus); commonly seen between 10 and 35 yrs of age, transmitted via saliva; incubation period is 5–15 days

**S/S:**
- Fever, malaise, fatigue, HA, lymphadenopathy (specifically posterior cervical chain), sore throat, anorexia, myalgias, hepatitis with hepatomegaly, splenomegaly, nausea, jaundice, photophobia, chest pain, dyspnea, pericarditis
- Other rare manifestations—maculopapular or petechial rash, exudative pharyngitis, tonsillitis, gingivitis

**Dx:**
- Labs—granulocytopenia → lymphocytic leukocytosis with atypical lymphocytes
- Mononucleosis spot test and heterophil test + within 4 wks of onset
- ↑ EBV titer
- CSF—↑ pressure, abnormal lymphocytes, protein (with neurologic involvement)
- ECG—abnormal T waves and prolonged PR intervals (with cardiologic involvement)

**Tx:**
- Supportive; there is no specific treatment
- Enforced bed rest until afebrile and restricted activity until hepato/splenomegaly resolves
- 5-day course of corticosteroids [methylprednisolone (Medrol dose pack)] may benefit severe cases

**Complications:** Secondary throat infection, rupture of spleen or HYPERSPLENISM, very rarely may result in BURKITT'S LYMPHOMA

## 13.10 MUMPS (EPIDEMIC PAROTITIS)

**Etiology:** An acute infection of the salivary glands, primarily the parotid glands, caused by *Paramyxovirus*

**S/S:** HA, anorexia, malaise, low-grade fever, pain and swelling of the parotid glands; may be one or both, may be one followed by the other 1–3 days later; orchitis

**Dx:** Clinical diagnosis

**Tx:**
- Symptomatic care—ASA, bed rest
- Must isolate patient until swelling subsides due to high level of contagiousness
- Treat complications as needed

**Complications:** Orchitis, oophoritis—can result in infertility; meningoencephalitis, pancreatitis, prostatitis, nephritis, myocarditis

## 13.11 NEONATAL SEPSIS

**Etiology:** Group B streptococci, *Escherichia coli, Listeria*

**S/S:** ↓ spontaneous activity, less vigorous sucking, respiratory distress, seizures, jaundice, vomiting, diarrhea, ABD distention, variable symptoms based on foci of infection, OM, OMPHALITIS, meningitis, septic arthritis, osteomyelitis, peritonitis

**Dx:**
- Labs—↑ WBCs, bands > 1,500, Gram's stain of BUFFY COAT—organisms (↑ if + blood Cx)
- LP—gross exam and cultures
- Blood and urine cultures

**Tx:** PCN or ampicillin plus aminoglycoside until cultures return, then adjust as needed

**Complications:** Meningitis with lifelong neurologic deficits, septic arthritis with permanent damage to joints, chronic osteomyelitis, death

## 13.12 OSTEOMYELITIS

**Etiology:** Infection of bone and marrow due to direct inoculation or hematogenous spread

**S/S:** Fever/chills, pain and point tenderness to involved area, redness, warmth, crepitus, purulent discharge, +/− abscess formation

**Dx:**
- Labs—leukocytosis with left shift
- X-ray—classic changes with lysis, periosteal changes
- Bone scan, CT, or MRI if x-ray is not diagnostic
- Needle or open biopsy to obtain culture prior to initiating antibiotic therapy

**Tx:**
- IV antibiotics for 6 weeks—start with empiric coverage until cultures return, then adjust as necessary [nafcillin, 1st generation cephalosporin, ampicillin/sulbactam (Unasyn), clindamycin, piperacillin (Zosyn), aminoglycoside]
- Surgical débridement—for all cases except vertebral due to discitis

**Complications:** Amputation, chronic osteomyelitis, sepsis

## 13.13 PERTUSSIS

**Etiology:** *Bordetella pertussis,* a Gram-negative coccobacillus; infection of the respiratory tract; transmitted via respiratory droplets; incubation period is 7–17 days

**S/S:** Three stages:
- Catarrhal stage—insidious onset, low-grade fever (if any), lacrimation, sneezing, coryza, anorexia, malaise, hacking night cough
- Paroxysmal stage—characteristic cough (rapid consecutive coughs followed by high-pitched inspiration), paroxysms may involve 5–15 consecutive coughs → few normal breaths → another paroxysm, copious viscous mucus, +/− vomiting during paroxysm; paroxysms triggered by stress, irritants, crying, sneezing, overdistention of ABD
- Convalescent stage—begins within 4 weeks; ↓ in frequency and severity of paroxysms of coughing

**Dx:** Labs—WBCs, 15,000–20,000/μL, 60%–80% lymphocytes; culture with Bordet-Gengou or other special medium to isolate

**Tx:**
- Erythromycin for 10 days may shorten the contagious period but is of little use during the paroxysmal stage
- For severe cases +/− corticosteroids for 4–6 days to ↓ intensity

**Complications:** Asphyxia, cerebral hemorrhage, pneumonia, atelectasis, interstitial and subcutaneous emphysema, pneumothorax

## 13.14  PINWORM INFECTION

**Etiology:** *Enterobius vermicularis,* 8- to 13-mm worm

**S/S:** Perianal pruritus, worse at night, insomnia, restlessness, enuresis, irritability

**Dx:** Confirmed by finding eggs on the perianal skin

**Tx:**
- Pyrantel pamoate or mebendazole
- All household members should be treated

**Complications:** Appendicitis, vulvovaginitis, urethritis, endometritis, salpingitis, pelvic granuloma, recurrent UTIs

## 13.15  SCARLET FEVER

**Etiology:** Due to erythrogenic toxin from group A streptococci

**S/S:** Fever, sore throat, tender cervical lymphadenopathy; diffuse erythematus, fine papular rash that blanches on pressure, rash may become petechial, fades to leave a fine desquamation, groin and axillae most intense, circumoral pallor, STRAW-BERRY TONGUE

**Dx:** Labs—leukocytosis with ↑ polymorphonuclear neutrophils; rapid antigen detection test + for group A strep

**Tx:**
- Benzathine PCN G or PCN V, if PCN allergy, erythromycin
- ASA, saline gargle PRN

**Complications:** Sinusitis, OM, mastoiditis, peritonsillar abscess, suppuration of cervical lymph nodes, rheumatic fever, glomerulonephritis

## 13.16 SEPSIS

**Etiology:**
- Systemic response to infection that compromises organ perfusion and may lead to multiorgan failure
- Pathogenesis—release of endotoxin → induces production of tumor necrosis factor and interleukins → triggers systemic inflammatory response and hypotension

**S/S:** Fevers/chills, hypotension, hyperventilation, hypothermia, mental status changes, tachycardia, cardiovascular collapse, ↓ SVR, normal pulmonary wedge pressure, local signs of infection depending on initial cause of infection, end-organ failure

**Dx:**
- Clinical diagnosis—hypotension that does not respond to fluid resuscitation
- Workup directed to find foci of infection—CXR, blood Cx, UA with C&S, Cx infected lines, LP

**Tx:**
- Antibiotics—directed by C&S
- DC indwelling catheters or devices if possible, drain any abscesses, I&D wounds as needed, hemodynamic support
- Supportive care—dialysis, continuous hemofiltration, mechanical ventilation, plasmapheresis

**Complications:** Death

## 13.17 SEPTIC ARTHRITIS

**Etiology:** Acute infection of the synovial space; usually due to hematogenous spread but may be due to direct inoculation

**S/S:** Pain, warmth, redness, and swelling of joint; fever/chills; refusal to move joint due to pain

**Dx:**
- Arthrocentesis—> 75K WBC; unless patient has been on antibiotics, organism usually noted on Gram's stain
- Labs—leukocytosis with left shift

**Tx:**
- Irrigation and débridement of joint is mandatory for all causes except *N. gonorrhoeae*
- IV antibiotics—definitive medication based on cultures, usually for 3 wks minimum

**Complications:** Arthritis, osteomyelitis, sepsis

## 13.18 SMALLPOX

**Etiology:** A variola virus; incubation period approximately 2 wks

**S/S:**
- Initial—high fever, fatigue, HA, backache, N/V
- Rash—usually follows onset by 2–3 days, prominent on face, extremities, and mucous membranes of mouth and nose; progresses from reddish macules → papules → pus-filled vesicles → crusting scabs
- All lesions in same stage of development, scabs fall off in 3–4 weeks

**Dx:** Clinical diagnosis, must distinguish from chickenpox

**Tx:**
- Strict isolation, no specific treatment (antivirals are in development stage)
- Supportive treatment—IV fluids, analgesics, antipyretics, antibiotics for secondary bacterial infections PRN
- Vaccine—available, but must be administered within 4 days of exposure (before rash develops); may prevent or diminish severity of illness in exposed individuals

**Complications:** Death

## 13.19 STREPTOCOCCAL PHARYNGITIS

**Etiology:** Group A beta-hemolytic streptococcus (*Strep. pyogenes*)

**S/S:** Sore throat; fever; HA; malaise; nausea; +/− ABD pain; enlarged, erythematous, exudative tonsils; cervical lymphadenopathy

**Dx:** Throat culture; rapid antigen detection test

**Tx:** 10-day course of oral PCN (erythromycin, azithromycin, or clindamycin for PCN allergy)

**Complications:** Scarlet fever, acute rheumatic fever, acute poststreptococcal glomerulonephritis

# CHAPTER 14

# Surgery

## 14.1 ACHALASIA: SURGICAL PERSPECTIVE

**Etiology:** Idiopathic neuromuscular disorder, causes esophageal dilatation and hypertrophy without organic stenosis; primary peristalsis is absent and cardioesophageal sphincter fails to relax with swallowing

**S/S:** Dysphagia, regurgitation of retained esophageal contents, +/− chest pain and esophageal spasms

**Dx:**
- X-rays—narrowing at cardia noted on barium swallow
- Fluoroscopy—weak, simultaneous, irregular, uncoordinated, or absent peristaltic waves
- Manometry—useful in confirming the diagnosis

**Tx:**
- Forceful dilation or direct surgical division of the cardia muscle fibers at the lower esophageal sphincter
- Ca channel blockers ↓ pressure in lower esophageal sphincter (not used often due to side effects)

**Complications:** Mucosal ulcerations, aspiration of regurgitated esophageal contents, malnutrition, squamous cell carcinoma

## 14.2 APPENDICITIS, ACUTE

**Etiology:**
- Obstruction of lumen of appendix by fecalith
- Pathogenesis—obstruction → distention of appendix and ↑ intraluminal pressure → venous engorgement and arterial ischemia → bacterial invasion of the wall → inflammation → appendicitis → necrosis → rupture → peritonitis

**S/S:** Periumbilical/epigastric pain (localizes to RLQ with time), anorexia, N/V, low-grade fever, RLQ TTP at McBurney's point, +/− rebound tenderness (rupture), ROVSING'S SIGN, PSOAS SIGN, OBTURATOR SIGN

**Dx:**
- Labs—leukocytosis
- ABD x-ray—+/− fecalith in RLQ
- US—diagnostic if positive, does not rule out if negative
- CT—good to assess for abscess

**Tx:** IV fluids, antibiotics for Gram-negative and anaerobic coverage; appendectomy is curative

**Complications:** Rupture, abscess formation, peritonitis, adhesions

## 14.3 ATELECTASIS

**Etiology:** Localized collapse of alveoli, develops with prolonged immobilization (during anesthesia, with forced bed rest)

**S/S:** Hypoxemia, bronchial breath sounds at the dependent portions of the lung

**Dx:** CXR—plate-like collapse of pulmonary parenchyma

**Tx:**
- Encourage deep breathing (inspiratory spirometry), cough, ambulation for most cases
- Severe—bronchoscopy, intubation, and mechanical ventilation

**Complications:** Pneumonia, cerebral edema (2° to severe hypoxemia), acute respiratory failure

## 14.4 BURNS

**Types:**
- 1°—superficial (sunburn)
- 2°—partial thickness (scalding/chemical)
- 3°—full thickness (flame)

**Etiology:** Damage to skin barrier, induces systemic immunosuppression, which predisposes to infection

**S/S:**
- 1°—painful erythema; dry skin without blistering; minimal or no edema
- 2°—moistened blisters; mottled gray or erythematous; extremely painful
- 3°—eschar formation; leathery or waxy appearance; dry, painless, pearly white or darkened lesions; hair easily removed; visibly thrombosed vessels
- Infected burns—↑ erythema or edema at margins; sudden separation of eschar from underlying tissue; fever; purulent drainage

**Dx:**
- Clinical diagnosis
- Rule of 9s—dorsal and ventral trunk, 18% each; arms, 9% each; legs, 18% each; perineum, 1%; head/neck, 9%

**Tx:** Immediate management: fluid maintenance and nutrition (initial 24 hr, crystalloid 4 mL/kg/% BSA); local wound care—topical agents to ↓ infectious burden on tissue; surgical excision of eschars with skin grafting; tetanus prophylaxis; pain control

**Complications:** Infection, pneumonia, pulmonary emboli, UTI, endocarditis, suppurative thrombophlebitis

## 14.5 CHOLECYSTITIS, ACUTE

**Etiology:** Inflammation of the gallbladder secondary to infection or obstruction; 95% are caused by gallstones

**S/S:** RUQ pain and tenderness to palpation, fever, N/V, right subscapular pain, +/− gallbladder palpable and painful, MURPHY'S SIGN

**Dx:**
- US—thickened gallbladder wall (> 3 mm); distended gallbladder; pericholecystic fluid; gallstones or ductal stones
- Labs—leukocytosis, ↑ LFTs, ↑ amylase, ↑ bilirubin, ↑ alkaline phosphatase

**Tx:** IV fluids; NG decompression; antibiotics; cholecystectomy (laparoscopic or open) is curative

**Complications:** Abscess formation, perforation, gallstone, ileus, formation of cholecystenteric fistula, recurrence (until removed)

## 14.6 DUMPING SYNDROME

**Etiology:** Any operation that impairs the ability of the stomach to regulate its rate of emptying

**S/S:** Two categories:
- Cardiovascular—palpitations, sweating, weakness, dyspnea, flushing, +/− syncope
- Gastrointestinal—nausea, ABD cramps, belching, vomiting, diarrhea

**Dx:** Clinical diagnosis based on symptoms in at-risk patients

**Tx:**
- Diet therapy—↓ jejunal osmolality (low carb, high fat, and protein)
- Surgical treatment is indicated for severe cases that do not respond to diet therapy

**Complications:** Malnutrition, postprandial hypoglycemia

## 14.7A ELECTROLYTE DISORDERS

**Causes:**

- ↑ Na+—fluid loss, steroid use, hypertonic fluid infusion
- ↓ Na+—TURP (due to copious bladder irrigation), adrenal insufficiency
- ↑ K+—acidosis, ↓ insulin, burns, crush injuries, leukocytosis
- ↓ K+—diarrhea, NG suction, vomiting, diuretics, Cushing's, burns
- ↑ $Ca^{2+}$—malignancy, disorders of bone, parathyroid or kidneys
- ↓ $Ca^{2+}$—acute pancreatitis, blood transfusions, renal failure, parathyroid resection
- ↑ $Mg^{2+}$—overuse of Mg supplements in renal failure patients
- ↓ $Mg^{2+}$—diarrhea, malabsorption, vomiting, alcoholism, aggressive diuresis
- ↑ Phos—usually iatrogenic; rhabdomyolysis, ↓ parathyroid, ↓ calcemia
- ↓ Phos—excessive IV glucose, ↑ parathyroidism, osmotic diuresis

**S/S:**

- ↑ Na+—lethargy, weakness, irritability; severe: seizures, coma
- ↓ Na+—severe: seizures, N/V, stupor or coma
- ↑ K+—heart block, ventricular fibrillation, asystole
- ↓ K+—ectopy, T-wave depression, prominent U waves, ventricular tachycardia
- ↑ $Ca^{2+}$—ALOC, muscle weakness, ileus, constipation, N/V, nephrolithiasis
- ↓ $Ca^{2+}$—paresthesias, tetany, seizures, weakness, ALOC
- ↑ $Mg^{2+}$—lethargy, weakness, ↓ DTRs, paralysis, ↓ BP and HR
- ↓ $Mg^{2+}$—torsades de pointes, ventricular fibrillation, atrial tachycardia, hyperreflexia, tetany
- ↑ Phos—soft tissue calcifications, heart block
- ↓ Phos—diffuse weakness, flaccid paralysis

*(continued)*

## 14.7B ELECTROLYTE DISORDERS, Continued

**Tx:**

- ↑ Na+—normal saline IV, correct 1/2 deficit in 1st 24 hr and rest over 2–3 days
- ↓ Na+—water restriction, hypertonic saline and loop diuretics
- ↑ K+—IV calcium gluconate, glucose and insulin, albuterol and loop diuretics
- ↓ K+—oral supplements +/− infusion < 10 mEq/hr, correct ↓ $Mg^{2+}$, +/− K+ sparing diuretics
- ↑ $Ca^{2+}$—calcium restriction, hydration and loop diuretics, calcitonin, pamidronate, dialysis
- ↓ $Ca^{2+}$—calcium gluconate, vitamin D supplementation
- ↑ $Mg^{2+}$—calcium gluconate, normal saline infusion with loop diuretics, +/− dialysis
- ↓ $Mg^{2+}$—magnesium sulfate
- ↑ Phos—↓ phosphorus intake, aluminum hydroxide, hydration and acetazolamide, +/− dialysis
- ↓ Phos—potassium phosphate or sodium phosphate

## 14.8 HEMORRHOIDS

**Types:**
- Internal—a plexus of superior hemorrhoidal veins above the mucocutaneous junction, covered by mucosa
- External—occur below the mucocutaneous junction in tissues beneath the anal epithelium

**Etiology:** Redundancy and enlargement of the vascular cushions of the normal anal venous plexus, occurs in all adults; when enlarged, become symptomatic; causes: straining for BM, chronic constipation, pregnancy, obesity, low-fiber diet, heavy lifting

**S/S:**
- Internal—rectal bleeding of bright red blood not mixed with stool, prolapse of the hemorrhoid with or without defecation, permanent prolapse → mucoid discharge and soiling of underwear
- External—pain +/− any of the above symptoms, palpable mass
- Graded—1st degree, bright red rectal bleeding, no prolapse; 2nd degree, prolapse with straining but reduce spontaneously; 3rd degree, prolapse with straining requiring manual reduction; 4th degree, fixed prolapse

**Dx:** Clinical diagnosis

**Tx:** Based on grade:
- 1st and 2nd degree—high-fiber diet, hydrophilic agents, +/− suppositories/ointments for symptomatic relief; for prolapse → reduce, bed rest, witch hazel compress +/− sitz baths +/− sclerotherapy
- 3rd and 4th degree—rubber-band ligation, cryosurgery, hemorrhoidectomy

**Complications:** Pain, thrombosis, recurrence, anemia

## 14.9 INFORMED CONSENT

**Requirements:**
- Description of the procedure, chances of success, risks and alternatives; must all be explained to pt in plain language that he or she can understand
- Signed consent form is only evidence that the process has occurred; it should be backed up by the physician's brief entry in the progress notes, including date and time

**Medical Emergencies:** Consent in a medical emergency is implied except when a **competent** adult refuses treatment; the patient's right to refuse treatment is not affected by the severity of the problem or the gravity of any potential consequences

**Doctrine of Proportionality:** Artificial life support should be initiated and maintained as long as it constitutes PROPORTIONATE TREATMENT

**Do Not Resuscitate (No Code) Orders:** Must be a written order in the patient's chart, supported by a written note from the attending physician, including the diagnosis and prognosis, wishes of the patient and family, consensus of the treatment team, and confirmation of the patient's competence

**Substitute Consent:** Consent from the next of kin in cases where the person in need of medical treatment is incapable of giving informed consent; order of intestate succession—spouse, adult child, parent, sibling

**Minor Consent:** Generally requires one parent; however, refusal by parents to consent in an emergency is subject to judicial review

## 14.10 INGUINAL HERNIA

**Etiology:**
- Congenital—due to a defect in the muscular layers of the abdomen
- Acquired—a result of a developed weakness of the transversalis fascia in Hesselbach's area
- Direct—hernial sac protrudes through the ABD wall in HESSELBACH'S TRIANGLE
- Indirect—hernial sac protrudes through the internal inguinal ring into the scrotum; sliding hernia is a type of indirect hernia where the wall of the viscus forms a portion of the wall of the hernial sac

**S/S:** Painless lump or mass in the groin, palpable mass with straining on PE

**Dx:** HERNIOGRAPHY, barium enema may reveal hernia

**Tx:** Surgical repair

**Complications:** Strangulated bowel, recurrent hernia

## 14.11 PANCREATIC PSEUDOCYST

**Etiology:** Encapsulated collections of fluid with high enzyme concentrations that arise from the pancreas, often secondary to severe acute pancreatitis or as a result of ductal obstruction and formation of a retention cyst that loses its epithelial lining as it grows beyond the confines of the gland

**S/S:** Palpable tender mass in the epigastrium, pain, fever, weight loss, tenderness, +/− jaundice

**Dx:**
- Labs—↑ serum amylase and leukocytosis, ↑ bilirubin
- CT—will reveal location and size of cyst
- ERCP—if significant abnormalities of the bile or pancreatic duct are suspected after CT

**Tx:** Three different surgical approaches can be used:
- Excision—most definitive treatment, recommended for posttraumatic cysts
- External drainage—best for critically ill patients; tube inserted into cyst and out through ABD wall
- Internal drainage—preferred treatment, cyst anastomosed to limb of jejunum, stomach, or duodenum

**Complications:** Infection, rupture, hemorrhage, recurrence

## 14.12 PANCREATITIS, ACUTE

**Definition:** Inappropriate activation of pancreatic enzyme precursors within the pancreas, leading to autodigestion, necrosis, edema, and hemorrhage

**Etiology:** Excessive alcohol intake; gallstones, biliary tract disease; trauma; viral; hypercalcemia; hypertriglyceridemia; drugs; ERCP

**S/S:**
- Steady, severe epigastric pain 1–4 hr after ingesting large meal or alcohol; ↓ pain when slumped forward, pain may radiate to back; N/V
- Severe disease—epigastric guarding, rebound TTP; fever; hypovolemia; tachycardia; shock; hypoxemia; ascites; ABD distention; left-sided pleural effusion; GREY-TURNER'S SIGN, CULLEN'S SIGN

**Dx:**
- CT/MRI with ↑ amylase is diagnostic
- Amylase—> 1,000 = biliary disease; 200–500 = ETOH pancreatitis
- X-ray—useful to assess for perforation or obstruction
- Labs—CBC = ↑ HCT, leukocytosis; LFTs ↑, hyperbilirubinemia

**Tx:** NPO, IV fluids, antibiotics, NG suction; pain control; treat any hyperglycemia or hypocalcemia; surgical indications: to relieve biliary or pancreatic duct obstruction, necrosis and sepsis

**Complications:** Shock, sepsis, DIC, ARDS, ATN, pancreatic abscess or pseudocyst, chronic pancreatitis

## 14.13 PERIRECTAL ABSCESS

**Etiology:** Bacterial invasion of the perirectal spaces, pathogens include *E. coli, Proteus vulgaris,* streptococci, staphylococci, and bacteroides

**S/S:** Pain, swelling, redness, tenderness, palpable tender mass on digital rectal exam

**Dx:** Clinical diagnosis

**Tx:** Incision and drainage followed by packing and healing by secondary intention

**Complications:** Persistent anorectal fistula, recurrence

## 14.14 PERITONITIS

**Etiology:**
- Inflammatory or suppurative response of the peritoneal lining to direct irritation due to perforation, inflammation, infection, or ischemic injuries of the GI or GU systems
- Secondary peritonitis—bacterial contamination originating from internal sources (within viscera) or from external sources (penetrating injury)

**S/S:** ABD pain, tenderness, guarding or rigidity, distention, free peritoneal air, ↓ bowel sounds, fever, chills, rigors, tachycardia, sweating, tachypnea, restlessness, dehydration, oliguria, disorientation, shock

**Dx:** Labs—CBC, ABG, PT/PTT, LFT, RFT; blood, urine, sputum, and peritoneal fluid for C&S

**Tx:**
- Fluid and electrolyte replacement, including blood transfusions if needed
- I&D peritoneum with aggressive debridement of all devitalized tissues
- Systemic antibiotics—start with empiric coverage of suspected pathogens until cultures return

**Complications:** Renal failure, liver failure, respiratory failure, cardiac failure, death

## 14.15 PREOPERATIVE EVALUATION

**Assessment:** An overall assessment of the patient's general health in order to identify significant abnormalities that might increase operative risk or adversely influence recovery should include the following:
- Comprehensive history and physical exam
- UA, CBC
- CXR
- All patients over 40 years—ECG, stool for occult blood, blood chemistry panel
- All significant complaints should be worked up with appropriate tests or consultations

**Operative Risk:** Specific factors affecting operative risk:
- Nutritional status—malnutrition leads to ↑ operative death rate
- Immune status—↑ risk of complications and death if impaired
- Pulmonary dysfunction—compromised pulmonary function pre-op ↑ risks of post-op complications
- Delayed wound healing—those with certain medical conditions are at ↑ risk of infection due to delayed healing
- Drug effects—allergies, sensitivities and incompatibilities, and adverse drug effects may lead to ↑ morbidity
- Pediatric or geriatric patients
- Obese patients—due to their risk of concomitant disease, these patients are at greater risk for complications

## 14.16 PSEUDOMEMBRANOUS ENTEROCOLITIS

**Etiology:** Acute inflammatory bowel disorder associated with antibiotic use, marked by exudative mucosal plaques; the most common cause is an overgrowth of *Clostridium difficile* due to antibiotic use

**S/S:** Loose stool → frank diarrhea, +/− colitis (bloody diarrhea, ABD pain, fever, leukocytosis), dehydration, hypotension, toxic megacolon, colonic perforation

**Dx:**
- Sigmoidoscopy to visualize the pseudomembranes within the distal colon
- Flat plate of the ABD—mucosal edema and abnormal haustral pattern
- Stool cultures confirm *C. difficile,* or assay for toxins

**Tx:**
- Stop any antibiotic being administered
- Colonic rest—clear liquids only until diarrhea resolves
- Metronidazole is the drug of choice, if unresponsive may change to oral vancomycin
- Severe cases may require hospitalization for IV hydration and antibiotics

**Complications:** Colonic perforation, severe dehydration, electrolyte imbalance, toxic megacolon

## 14.17 RUPTURED SPLEEN

**Etiology:**
- Disruption of the parenchyma, capsule, or blood supply of the spleen; most common major injury from blunt ABD trauma but may occur spontaneously in an enlarged, diseased spleen (malaria, mononucleosis, lymphoma, leukemia, typhoid fever)
- Delayed rupture—rupture due to relatively minor insult, usually days to weeks after the event

**S/S:**
- Severe hypovolemic shock to no symptoms; usually a history of trauma, generalized ABD pain (↑ LUQ), +/− KEHR'S SIGN
- P/E—TTP of ABD, +/− ABD distention, splenic dullness to percussion, +/− mass to LUQ

**Dx:**
- Labs—↓ hematocrit over time, WBC ↑ with left shift
- Flat plate of ABD—+/− Fx ribs, splenomegaly, displacement of gastric bubble, serrated appearance to greater curvature of stomach
- CT—demonstrate splenic enlargement and intraparenchymal hematomas

**Tx:**
- Laparotomy is usually indicated (75% of time)
- Nonoperative treatment is indicated if the patient meets the following criteria: (1) injury due to blunt trauma (not penetrating); (2) no other surgical injuries; (3) patient is hemodynamically stable; (4) total transfusion requirements do not exceed 2 units; (5) no significant increase in size of lesion within the spleen on serial CT scans

**Complications:** Hypovolemia, death

## 14.18 SUPERIOR VENA CAVA SYNDROME

**Etiology:** Superior vena cava obstruction due to malignant tumors (80%–90%), benign tumors, metastatic tumors or other space-occupying lesions in the mediastinum, including thrombosis

**S/S:**
- Puffiness of the face, arms, shoulders; blue or purple discoloration of the skin
- CNS—HA, nausea, dizziness, vomiting, distortion of vision, drowsiness, stupor, and convulsions
- Pulmonary system—cough, hoarseness, dyspnea, made worse with supine or bent-over position
- Symptoms may develop slowly or suddenly

**Dx:**
- CXR—may show RUL lesion or R paratracheal mass
- Aortography—if aneurysm suspected
- CT scan with contrast is usually diagnostic

**Tx:**
- If caused by cancer—diuretics, fluid restriction, and prompt radiation therapy
- If of other cause—surgical excision of the compressing mass, bypass procedures for thrombotic cases

**Complications:** Cerebral edema, asphyxiation, death

## 14.19 TESTICULAR TORSION

**Etiology:** Most commonly due to a lack of the posterior attachment to the tunica vaginalis; this allows the testis to rotate around the spermatic cord

**S/S:** Acute onset of unilateral scrotal pain, N/V, swollen TTP testicle, absent cremasteric reflex on the affected side, testicle has a transverse lie

**Dx:**
- Clinical diagnosis
- US may be used to assess flow to the testicle if the patient presents early
- DO NOT delay treatment to obtain tests

**Tx:**
- Emergent surgical exploration and decompression is necessary to save the testicle
- Must perform B/L orchiopexy to prevent torsional damage to other testicle
- If testicle is necrotic, must be removed to ↓ chance of infertility

**Complications:** Infertility, recurrence

## 14.20  WHOLE BLOOD TRANSFUSIONS

**Banked Blood:**
- Whole blood can be stored for up to 35 days
- ↑ Lactic acid, inorganic phosphate, ammonia, and potassium in stored blood, usually will not be significant except for those patients with renal or hepatic impairment
- Platelets, factors V and VIII deteriorate; after 2 days of refrigerated storage, blood is basically devoid of viable platelets (massive transfusions = thrombocytopenia)

**Serologic Considerations:**
- Emergency transfusions—type-specific packed red cells or whole blood preferred
- O-negative packed red cells may be given to any patient (universal donor)
- Elective transfusions—for maximal compatibility → antibody screen and cross-match, process takes about 1 hr

**Amount for Transfusion:**
- Adults—1 unit of packed red cells, ↑ hemoglobin by 1 g/dL and hematocrit by 3% for the average adult (70 kg)
- Children—over 25 kg = 500 mL; under 25 kg = 20 mL/kg
- Premie—10 mL/kg

**Rate of Transfusion:** Generally 500 mL should be given in 1–2 hr; in patients with heart disease, allow 2–3 hr

**Complications:** Fever, allergic reactions, transmission of diseases (hepatitis, AIDS), bacterial contamination, hemolytic reactions, circulatory complications due to too rapid transfusion, death

## 14.21  WOUND INFECTION, POSTOPERATIVE

**Etiology:** Results from bacterial contamination during or after a surgical procedure; usually confined to subcutaneous tissues

**S/S:** Fever, redness, pain, +/− purulent drainage from wound, +/− fluctuance or induration

**Dx:** Clinical diagnosis, identify pathogen by culture of discharge

**Tx:**
- Irrigation and débridement
- Antibiotics

**Complications:** ↑ morbidity rate from underlying medical conditions, multisystem failure, sepsis, osteomyelitis, amputations

# CHAPTER 15

# Pharmacology

## 15.1A ANTIARRHYTHMICS

**Mechanisms and Sites of Action:**
- Class I—sodium channel antagonists; ↓ upstroke and amplitude of cardiac action potential = ↓ conduction velocity in injured tissues
  - Class IA—have anticholinergic actions
  - Class IB—act on sodium channels in ventricle with minimal effects on nodal or conduction tissues
  - Class IC—slows conduction velocity by slowing initial depolarization

**Primary Action(s) and Use(s):**
- Class I—**prolonged action potential → prolonged QT segment**
  - Class IA—effective for both atrial and ventricular arrhythmias; may ↑ ventricular response in atrial fibrillation/flutter
  - Class IB—major effect is in suppressing arrhythmias associated with depolarization; shortens action potential duration = ↓ risk for reentrant arrhythmias
  - Class IC—principal use is for ventricular arrhythmias; also effective at suppressing PVCs and ↓ ventricular response to atrial fibrillation/flutter

**Side Effects and Toxicity:**
- Class I—↑ risk of reentrant arrhythmias
  - Class IA—renal elimination inhibited by high digoxin levels; high levels can cause complete AV block
  - Class IB—primarily CNS = seizures, drowsiness, paresthesias
  - Class IC—may ↑ risk of death due to proarrhythmogenic effects

**Representative Drugs:** Class IA, procainamide; class IB, lidocaine; class IC, flecainide

*(continued)*

## 15.1B ANTIARRHYTHMICS, Continued

**Mechanisms and Sites of Action:**
- Class II—beta blockers: adrenolytic, inhibit postsynaptic beta receptors
- Class III—prolong the action potential duration without altering initial depolarization of the resting membrane potential
- Class IV—calcium channel blockers (nondihydropyridines); **predominant effect is on SA and AV nodes**
- Adenosine—binds to adenosine receptors in AV node, causes immediate cessation of nodal reentrant tachycardia
- Magnesium—shortens QT duration

**Primary Action(s) and Use(s):**
- Class II—hypertension, myocardial ischemia, heart failure, rate control in tachycardias
- Class III—principal use is intractable ventricular tachycardia and fibrillation
- Class IV—can abort reentrant tachycardias and slow ventricular rate in atrial fibrillation and flutter
- Adenosine—1st-line drug for supraventricular tachycardia
- Magnesium—1st-line drug for torsade de pointes

**Side Effects and Toxicity:**
- Class II—bronchospasm, worsen heart block, cause hypoglycemia
- Class III, amiodarone—pulmonary fibrosis, hyper- or hypothyroid, hepatic necrosis/fibrosis
- Class IV—may worsen heart failure due to negative inotropic actions; do not use with beta-blockers
- Adenosine—marked flushing and chest burning, may induce high-grade heart block

**Representative Drugs:** Class II—propranolol; class III—amiodarone; class IV—verapamil; miscellaneous—adenosine, magnesium

## 15.2 DIURETICS

**Mechanisms and Sites of Action:**
- Thiazide—inhibit sodium chloride resorption in the distal convoluted tubules
- Loop—inhibit sodium chloride resorption in the ascending limb of the loop of Henle
- Potassium-sparing—act in the cortical collecting tubule and late distal tubule
- Carbonic anhydrase inhibitors—work in the proximal tubule
- Osmotic—stay in the tubules and draw water into the tubules promoting diuresis

**Primary Action(s) and Use(s):**
- Thiazide—1st-line along with beta blockers for essential hypertension
- Loop—1° used for diuresis of water in patients with significant volume overload
- Potassium-sparing—1° use is in combination with other diuretics to prevent hypokalemia
- Carbonic anhydrase inhibitors—1° use is in eyedrops to treat glaucoma and to prevent and treat altitude sickness
- Osmotic—1° use is for elevated intracranial pressure

**Side Effects and Toxicity:**
- Thiazide—enhance calcium absorption, inhibit uric acid secretion, contain sulfa moieties (sulfa allergen)
- Loop—inhibit excretion of uric acid, cause loss of calcium in urine, contain sulfa moieties
- Potassium-sparing—antagonize effects of aldosterone, may cause hyperkalemia
- Carbonic anhydrase inhibitors—hyperchloremic metabolic acidosis and massive potassium wasting
- Osmotic—dehydration and vascular collapse

**Representative Drugs:** Thiazide = hydrochlorothiazide; loop = furosemide; potassium-sparing = spironolactone; carbonic anhydrase inhibitor = acetazolamide; osmotic = mannitol

## 15.3 INOTROPES

**Mechanisms and Sites of Action:**
- Digoxin—prevents uptake of potassium and export of sodium from the cell
- Milrinone and amrinone—phosphodiesterase inhibitors
- Dopamine—binds to alpha$_1$ receptors in periphery and beta$_1$ receptors on the heart
- Dobutamine—binds to beta$_1$ receptors on the heart

**Primary Action(s) and Use(s):**
- Digoxin—leads to ↑ intracellular calcium = ↑ myocardial contractility → ↑ cardiac output; also has cholinomimetic effects on SA and AV nodes = slowed ventricular response to atrial fibrillation
- Milrinone and amrinone—↑ muscle contraction and ↑ heart rate; **only used acutely for cardiogenic shock**
- Dopamine—↑ systemic vascular resistance, heart rate, and contractility; **1° use = hypotension 2° to low SVR;** at low doses causes renal vasodilation and ↑ renal perfusion
- Dobutamine—↑ contractility → ↑ cardiac output; **1st-line drug for acute severe heart failure**

**Side Effects and Toxicity:**
- Digoxin—arrhythmias, PVCs, slows cardiac conduction, SVT, ventricular tachycardia, CNS and GI toxicity; renal failure prolongs dig half-life; hypokalemia induces dig toxicity
- Milrinone and amrinone—marked increase in myocardial oxygen consumption
- Dopamine—increased myocardial oxygen consumption
- Dobutamine—autonomic reflex decreases systemic vascular resistance; cannot be used alone in cardiogenic shock, must be combined with vasoconstrictors

## 15.4A VASODILATORS

**Mechanisms and Sites of Action:**
- Nitrates—steadily releases nitric oxide into the vasculature; effects on both arteries and veins
- Calcium channel blockers—prevent influx of calcium, work on both vascular and cardiac muscle
- Hydralazine—causes direct arteriolar vasodilation
- Minoxidil—causes closure of calcium channels by opening the potassium channel on smooth muscle
- ACE inhibitors—convert angiotensin I to angiotensin II = potent vasoconstriction due to catecholamine release; also block the degradation of bradykinin = direct vasodilation
- Angiotensin II receptor antagonists (ATRAs)—block the binding of angiotensin II to its receptor

**Primary Action(s) and Use(s):**
- Nitrates—$\downarrow$ myocardial oxygen demand, causes dilation of both arteries and veins; 1° indication is acute ischemic chest pain and hypertensive crisis
- Calcium channel blockers—2 general classes:
  - Dihydropyridines (all end in "-ine")—affect vasculature more than cardiac muscle; 1° indication HTN
  - Nondihydropyridines—equal or greater effect on cardiac muscle; 1° indication is arrhythmia
- Hydralazine—$\downarrow$ afterload without affecting preload; 2nd-line drug for heart failure; proven $\downarrow$ mortality when combined with isosorbide dinitrate
- Minoxidil—severe, refractory hypertension is only indication; topical version—hair-growth stimulator
- ACE inhibitors—1st-line drug for low ejection fraction, post-MI, diabetic patients and patients with proteinuria (proven to $\downarrow$ mortality in all the above)
- ATRAs—share many of the properties of ACE inhibitors but do not cause cough

*(continued)*

## 15.4B VASODILATORS, Continued

**Side Effects and Toxicity:**
- Nitrates—prolonged use can lead to cyanide toxicity (nitroprusside)
- Calcium channel blockers—autonomic reflex tachycardia; must use beta blockers concurrently (dihydropyridines); avoid in heart failure; do not give beta blockers concurrently, may cause complete heart block (nondihydropyridine)
- Hydralazine—reflex tachycardia; must use beta blocker concurrently
- Minoxidil—reflex tachycardia and fluid retention; must use beta blocker and diuretic concurrently
- ACE inhibitors—chronic cough, angioedema, hyperkalemia, $\uparrow$ creatinine
- ATRAs—$\uparrow$ creatinine, hyperkalemia

**Representative Drugs:**
- Nitrates—nitroglycerin, isosorbide dinitrate, nitroprusside
- Calcium channel blockers—verapamil, diltiazem
- ACE inhibitors—captopril, enalapril, benazepril, lisinopril, fosinopril, ramipril
- Angiotensin II receptor antagonists—losartan, candesartan, irbesartan, valsartan

## 15.5 AUTONOMIC MEDICATIONS

**Types:**

*Cholinomimetics:* Two classes:
- Direct receptor agonists
- Inhibitors of acetylcholinesterase

*Cholinolytics:* Three types:
- Muscarinic receptor antagonists
- Ganglionic blockers
- Neuromuscular blockers

*Sympathomimetics (adrenomimetics):* Three classes:
- Direct agonists
- Indirect agonists
- Mixed agonists

*Sympatholytics (adrenolytics):* Three classes:
- Presynaptic adrenergic inhibitors
- Postsynaptic alpha-receptor blockers
- Postsynaptic beta-receptor blockers

**Mechanisms and Sites of Action:**

*Cholinomimetics*
- Direct receptor agonists—chemically resistant to degradation by acetylcholinesterase
- Acetylcholinesterase inhibitors—competitive reversible inhibitors, carbamates, irreversible inhibitors

*Cholinolytics*
- Muscarinic receptor antagonists—↓ smooth muscle contraction in visceral smooth muscle
- Ganglionic blockers—affect peripheral parasympathetic nerve synapses, sympathetic and parasympathetic ganglionic synapses
- Neuromuscular blocking agents—more potent at blocking skeletal muscle nicotinic receptors than autonomic receptors; 2 subtypes, depolarizing and nondepolarizing

*Sympathomimetics*
- Direct agonists—bind to alpha or beta receptors
- Indirect agonists—↑ level of norepinephrine in synaptic cleft
- Mixed agonists—bind to receptors and ↑ level of norepinephrine in synaptic cleft

*Sympatholytics*
- Inhibitors of presynaptic signaling—inhibit synthesis, storage, or release of catecholamines
- Alpha blockers—antagonize $alpha_1$ and/or $alpha_2$ receptors
- Beta blockers—antagonize $beta_1$ and/or $beta_2$ receptors

## 15.6 AUTONOMIC MEDICATIONS: CHOLINOMIMETICS AND CHOLINOLYTICS

**Primary Action(s) and Use(s):**

*Cholinomimetics*
- Bethanechol—stimulates urination in patients with neurogenic bladder
- Pilocarpine—topical eyedrop to ↓ pressure in glaucoma
- Edrophonium—reversible inhibitor, short-acting; used to Dx myasthenia gravis
- Neostigmine/pyridostigmine—carbamate, longer-acting; used to Tx myasthenia gravis
- Physostigmine—carbamate, used in eyedrops to ↓ intraocular pressure in glaucoma

*Cholinolytics*
- Atropine—used to Tx bradycardia and heart block, also to reverse cholinergic poisoning
- Benztropine/trihexyphenidyl—↓ cholinergic signaling; helps restore the cholinergic/dopaminergic balance in brain; Tx Parkinson's disease
- Cyclopentolate—muscarinic antagonist; used in eyedrops to allow funduscopic examination

- Ipratropium—bronchodilation; used as inhaler to treat asthma
- Oxybutynin—urinary stimulant; used as Tx for neurogenic bladder
- Scopolamine—may be used orally or topically as Tx for motion sickness
- Trimethaphan—used for HTN crisis, short half-life allows rapid titration to affect rapid BP changes

**Side Effects and Toxicity:**

*Cholinomimetics:* Organophosphate poisoning—hypersecretion of saliva and mucus, bronchospasm, bradycardia, vomiting, diarrhea

*Cholinolytics:*
- Muscarinic antagonists—"dry as a bone, mad as a hatter, hot as a hare, blind as a bat"
- Ganglionic blockers—tachycardia, hypotension, constipation, urinary retention, ↓ accommodation
- Neuromuscular blocking agents—hyperkalemia 2° to muscle fasciculations (depolarizing agents)

## 15.7A AUTONOMIC MEDICATIONS: SYMPATHOMIMETICS

**Primary Action(s) and Use(s):**

*Direct Agonists*

- Norepinephrine—profound alpha$_1$-mediated vasoconstriction = ↑ systolic and diastolic B/P
  - Side effects: normotensive host = reflex bradycardia; hypotensive host = tachycardia
- Epinephrine—↑ myocardial contractility and heart rate; **1st-line drug for anaphylactic shock and cardiac resuscitation**
  - Side effects—normotensive host = widening of pulse pressure; hypotensive host = vasoconstriction, bronchodilation, and ↑ contractility and heart rate
- Isoproterenol—↑ heart rate and contractility and ↓ SVR = marked widening of pulse pressure
  - Side effects—slight ↓ overall mean arterial pressure
- Dopamine—↑ vasoconstriction = ↑ B/P; ↑ contractility = ↑HR; **1st-line drug for most clinical conditions requiring use of a pressor**
  - Side effects—pts with poor ejection fractions may not respond as well
- Dobutamine—↑ contractility and HR; **drug of choice in heart failure**
  - Side effects—reflexive vasodilation
- Phenylephrine—vasoconstriction = ↑ B/P; **useful for patients with tachycardia or ischemia;** eyedrops stimulate mydriasis for funduscopic exam; used as nasal decongestant—vasoconstriction of nasal vasculature = ↓ mucosal edema
- Albuterol—used as inhaled bronchodilators for asthma
  - Side effects—systemic absorption = vasodilation and reflex tachycardia

*(continued)*

## 15.7B AUTONOMIC MEDICATIONS: SYMPATHOMIMETICS, Continued

**Primary Action(s) and Use(s):**

*Indirect Agonists*

- Tyramine—causes release of stored norepinephrine; mimics direct administration of norepinephrine
  - Side effect—severe ↑ B/P in patients taking MAO inhibitors
- Amphetamine—stimulates release of catecholamines
  - Side effects—potent CNS effects
- Pseudoephedrine—dominant effect is to stimulate release of catecholamines, also is a weak direct agonist; predominantly found in nasal decongestants and eyedrops for funduscopic examinations
  - Side effects—hypertension
- Cocaine—inhibits reuptake of catecholamines in the synaptic cleft;
  - Side effects—prolonged stimulation of the CNS adrenergic neurons
- MAO inhibitors—anticholinergic effects and serotonin-stimulatory effects; minimal pressor effects unless mixed with high doses of tyramine

## 15.8A AUTONOMIC MEDICATIONS: SYMPATHOLYTICS

**Beta Blockers:**
- Inhibitors of postsynaptic beta receptors
- Proven to ↓ mortality in hypertension
- ↓ mortality in myocardial ischemia
- ↓ mortality in heart failure
- **1° indication is HTN, myocardial ischemia, heart failure, tachyarrhythmias, and control of HTN in aortic dissection**
- 2° uses for migraine HA, thyroid storm, tremor, and performance anxiety

**Primary Action(s) and Use(s):**
- Acebutolol—$beta_1$-selective, **primary use HTN**
- Atenolol—$beta_1$-selective, **primary use HTN**
- Betaxolol—most highly $beta_1$-selective of all available drugs, **primary use HTN**
- Metoprolol—$beta_1$-selective; used in HTN, acute ischemia, heart failure
- Bisoprolol—$beta_1$-selective use in HTN and heart failure

- Esmolol—$beta_1$-selective, extremely short-acting, **1st line drug for acute aortic dissection;** other uses in HTN emergency or acute SVT refractory to other medications
- Propranolol—nonselective beta blocker, short acting, highly lipophilic → causes more CNS effects than other medications; used for control of essential tremor or performance anxiety disorder; also used as prophylaxis to prevent variceal bleeding in patients with portal hypertension
- Timolol—nonselective beta blocker, **major use is in eyedrops for glaucoma**
- Labetalol—nonselective adrenergic inhibitor, **major use in HTN, HTN emergency, aortic dissection**
- Carvedilol—nonselective adrenergic inhibitor, **1st-line drug for heart failure;** 1st beta blocker proven to ↓ mortality in HF; only beta blocker proven to ↓ mortality in severe (class IV) HF

*(continued)*

## 15.8B AUTONOMIC MEDICATIONS: SYMPATHOLYTICS, Continued

**Beta Blockers:**
**Side Effects and Toxicity:**
- All beta blockers have potential to induce bronchospasm; worsen or precipitate heart block; inhibit insulin release and thus induce frank diabetes or worsen glycemic control in impaired glucose tolerance; cause hypoglycemia in diabetics by blunting normal neurologic response to hypoglycemia and inhibiting glycogenolysis; acutely worsening heart failure in CHF if patients are fluid-overloaded
- Minor toxic effects—rash, fever, sedation, sleep disturbances, depression
- Major adverse effects:
  ○ May worsen severe peripheral vascular disease or vasospastic disorders; in patients with abnormal myocardial function, even small doses may provoke severe cardiac failure
  ○ Severe hypotension, bradycardia, CHF, and cardiac conduction abnormalities are possible if given with calcium channel blockers
  ○ Must taper off medications after chronic use

*(continued)*

## 15.8C AUTONOMIC MEDICATIONS: SYMPATHOLYTICS, Continued

**Inhibitors of Presynaptic Adrenergic Signaling:**
- Rarely used because of CNS depression and other toxicity
- **The only 1° use is as an antihypertensive in pregnant women**

**Primary Action(s) and Use(s):**
*Clonidine*
- Inhibits release of norepinephrine from presynaptic terminals
- Causes vasodilation by suppressing norepinephrine-mediated constriction; no reflex tachycardia
- **1° indication is refractory hypertension with renal failure or patients withdrawing from drugs**
- Side effects—CNS depression, fatigue, dry mouth

*Methyldopa*
- Partial agonist-antagonist of alpha$_1$ receptors; inhibits norepinephrine synthesis
- Acts as an alternative substrate for dopamine decarboxylase

- **Only 1st-line indication is hypertension in pregnancy**
- Side effects—CNS depression, drug-induced lupus

*Metyrosine*
- Competitively inhibits tyrosine hydroxylase = blockage of norepinephrine synthesis
- **Limited clinical usefulness**
- Side effects—severe CNS depression

*Guanethidine:* Four effects:
- Reserpine-like block of uptake into synaptic vesicles (**dominant effect**)
- Inhibits catecholamine release from presynaptic terminus
- Presynaptic depletion of norepinephrine (causes initial ↑ BP followed by ↓)
- Exerts a cocaine-like blockade of norepinephrine re-uptake into the presynaptic nerve terminus; contributes to an initial ↑ BP
- **Limited clinical usefulness**

*(continued)*

## 15.8D AUTONOMIC MEDICATIONS: SYMPATHOLYTICS, Continued

**Alpha Blockers:**
- Inhibitors of postsynaptic alpha$_1$ receptors
- Usefulness is limited due to a marked reflex tachycardia

**Primary Action(s) and Use(s):**
*Phentolamine*
- Potent vasodilator—↓ BP
- **1° indication is pheochromocytoma-induced hypertension**
- Side effects—severe reflex tachycardia and palpitations, nasal congestion, miosis, ↓ ejaculation, diarrhea

*Prazosin, Terazosin, Doxazocin*
- Selective alpha$_1$ antagonists
- **1° use is BPH and hypertension in the same patient**
- Side effects—prominent orthostatic hypotension, moderate reflex tachycardia

*Tolazoline*
- Similar to phentolamine but less potent and better absorbed from GI tract
- **1° indication is peripheral vasospastic disease and pulmonary HTN in newborn with respiratory distress syndrome**
- Side effects—tachycardia, diarrhea

*Ergot Derivatives*
- Vasoconstriction
- **1° use is Tx of migraine** (ergotamine)

SECTION B
## Pulmonary System Medications

## 15.9 BRONCHODILATORS

**Mechanisms and Sites of Action:**
- Sympathomimetics—adrenergic agents (beta$_2$), inhibit mediator release
- Cholinolytics—muscarinic antagonists—competitively inhibit the effect of acetylcholine → block contraction of airway smooth muscle and excess secretions

**Primary Action(s) and Use(s):**
- Sympathomimetics—smooth muscle relaxation in the bronchioles is pure beta$_2$; nonselective beta effects include ↑ contractility and HR, vasodilation, ↓ BP; used for asthma delivered via IV, SQ, PO, inhaled
- Cholinolytics—bronchodilation and ↓ mucous secretion; used for asthma and emphysema

**Side Effects and Toxicity:**
- Sympathomimetics—skeletal muscle tremor, vasodilation and reflex tachycardia
- Cholinolytics—urinary retention, tachycardia, loss of visual accommodation, agitation

**Representative Drugs:**
- Sympathomimetics—epinephrine, isoproterenol, salmeterol
- Cholinolytics—ipratropium bromide

## 15.10A  ANTIASTHMATICS

**Mechanisms and Sites of Action:**
- Cromolyn sodium—prevents antigen-induced release of histamine and other mediators of anaphylaxis from sensitized mast cells
- Corticosteroids—precise mechanism unknown, possibly potentiates the effects of beta-receptor agonists and modifies inflammatory response in airways
- Methotrexate—potent anti-inflammatory
- Gold—↓ bronchial reactivity
- Theophylline—inhibits the enzyme phosphodiesterase

**Primary Action(s) and Use(s):**
- Cromolyn sodium—Tx for exercise- and ASA-induced bronchoconstriction, prophylactic for perennial asthma or seasonal allergic asthma
- Corticosteroid—potent anti-inflammatory, works to ↓ airway constriction due to inflammation
- Methotrexate—used to taper dose of steroid required for steroid-dependent asthmatics
- Gold—↓ symptoms and dose of steroid in severe asthmatics
- Theophylline—severe asthma, COPD

*(continued)*

## 15.10B  ANTIASTHMATICS, Continued

**Side Effects and Toxicity:**
- Cromolyn sodium—throat irritation, cough, mouth dryness, chest tightness, wheezing, myositis, gastroenteritis, reversible dermatitis
- Corticosteroids—↑ risk of infection, peptic ulcer/GI hemorrhage, psychosis, AVN, cataracts, severe osteoporosis, Cushing's syndrome, adrenal insufficiency with sudden withdrawal
- Methotrexate—dose-related hepatic fibrosis, GI and bone marrow toxicity
- Gold—severe skin rash, hepatic/renal damage, blood dyscrasias
- Theophylline—↑ HR, PVCs, anorexia, N/V, ABD discomfort, lowers seizure threshold

**Representative Drugs:**
- Cromolyn sodium
- Corticosteroids—prednisone, triamcinolone, beclomethasone, flunisolide, fluticasone
- Methotrexate
- Gold
- Theophylline

# SECTION C
## *Gastrointestinal System Medications*

### 15.11A  ANTACIDS

**Mechanisms and Sites of Action:**
- $H_2$ blockers—suppress acid production
- Proton-pump inhibitors—inhibit gastric parietal cell proton pump
- Direct antacids—neutralize acid directly by binding with the hydrochloric acid in the stomach
- Metoclopramide—potent dopamine antagonist with cholinomimetic properties
- Sucralfate, bismuth subsalicylate (Pepto-Bismol)—act as physical barriers to acid as it binds to stomach lining

**Primary Action(s) and Use(s):**
- $H_2$ blockers—1st-line Tx for gastric and duodenal ulcers and hypersecretory states
- Proton-pump inhibitors—1st-line therapy for ulcers, bleeding gastritis, Barrett's esophagitis
- Direct antacids—used for symptomatic relief of indigestion
- Metoclopramide—acts as a gut stimulant in cases of hypomotility; 1° indication = diabetic gastroparesis
- Sucralfate, bismuth subsalicylate (Pepto-Bismol)—binds to ulcer tissue in the stomach; 1° indication is peptic ulcer disease

*(continued)*

## 15.11B ANTACIDS, Continued

**Side Effects and Toxicity:**
- $H_2$ blockers—drug-induced thrombocytopenia, confusional states in elderly, +/− gynecomastia, male sexual dysfunction
- Proton-pump inhibitors—HA, diarrhea, ABD pain, constipation, flatulence, monitor warfarin (Coumadin) and digoxin levels
- Direct antacids—change in bowel habits, alkalosis in patients with renal impairment
- Metoclopramide—somnolence, nervousness, dystonic reactions, parkinsonism, tardive dyskinesia, +/− menstrual disorders, galactorrhea
- Bismuth subsalicylate (Pepto-Bismol)—change in stool color and consistency

**Representative Drugs:**
- $H_2$ blockers—cimetidine, ranitidine
- Proton-pump inhibitors—omeprazole, lansoprazole, esomeprazole, pantoprazole
- Direct antacids—calcium carbonate (TUMS), magnesium salts, magnesium hydroxide
- Metoclopramide
- Bismuth subsalicylate (Pepto-Bismol)

## 15.12 ANTIDIARRHEALS

**Mechanisms and Sites of Action:**
- Bismuth subsalicylate (Kaopectate)—adsorbs compounds from solution → binds to potential intestinal toxins
- Diphenoxylate and atropine (Lomotil)—in the large intestine, propulsive peristaltic waves are ↓ and tone is ↑ resulting in delay in passage of fecal mass → ↑ water absorption (constipation)
- Loperamide (Imodium)—chemically related to haloperidol; mechanism same as that of Lomotil
- Bismuth subsalicylate (Pepto-Bismol)—↓ fluid secretion into the bowel, +/− antimicrobial properties (*Clostridium difficile*)

**Primary Action(s) and Use(s):**
- Kaopectate—physical coating of mucosa, absorbs water out of stool; 1° indication = noninfectious diarrhea
- Lomotil—antidiarrheal and antispasmodic; 1° indication = moderate to severe diarrhea
- Imodium—same as Lomotil
- Pepto-Bismol—1° indication = mild to moderate diarrhea with or without N/V, gas

**Side Effects and Toxicity:**
- Kaopectate—constipation
- Lomotil and Imodium—worsening inflammation, bowel perforation, toxic megacolon
- Pepto-Bismol—constipation, stool color change

## 15.13 ANTIEMETICS

**Mechanisms and Sites of Action:** All work in the CNS chemoreceptor trigger zone:
- Phenothiazines—dopamine antagonists ($D_2$)
- Metoclopramide—dopamine ($D_2$) and serotonin receptor ($5\text{-}HT_3$) antagonist
- Ondansetron and granisetron—serotonin receptor ($5\text{-}HT_3$) antagonists
- Muscarinic antagonists—atropine, scopolamine, diphenhydramine

**Primary Action(s) and Use(s):**
- Phenothiazines—1° indication = N/V, 1st-line Tx for hospitalized patients
- Metoclopramide—1° indication = nausea with dysmotility (diabetic gastroparesis), and chemotherapy N/V
- Ondansetron and granisetron—1° indication = nausea associated with chemotherapy
- Atropine—1° indication = cholinergic toxicity
- Scopolamine and diphenhydramine—1° indication = motion sickness

**Side Effects and Toxicity:**
- Phenothiazines—urinary retention, orthostatic hypotension, impaired ejaculation, confusional states at very high doses; toxicity—agranulocytosis, cholestatic jaundice, skin eruptions
- Metoclopramide—somnolence, nervousness, dystonic reactions, parkinsonism, tardive dyskinesia, ↑ pituitary prolactin release, galactorrhea, menstrual disorders
- Muscarinic antagonists—drowsiness, dry mouth, excitement, agitation, hallucinations, coma

**Representative Drugs:**
- Phenothiazines—prochlorperazine (compazine)
- Muscarinic antagonists—scopolamine

## 15.14 ANTICONSTIPATION MEDICATIONS

**Mechanisms and Sites of Action:**
- Osmotic laxatives—hypertonic solutions → draw fluid into the bowel
- Bulk laxatives—nondigestible fiber → forms a gel within the large intestine, stimulates peristaltic activity
- Mucosal stimulants—stimulate peristalsis within the colon
- Stool softeners—detergents → allow water to penetrate stool

**Primary Action(s) and Use(s):** All are 1° used for constipation

**Side Effects and Toxicity:** With prolonged use, patient may become dependent on any type of laxative

**Representative Drugs:**
- Osmotic laxatives—magnesium citrate and magnesium hydroxide, lactulose
- Bulk laxatives—hydrophilic colloids, bran, psyllium seed
- Mucosal stimulants—cascara, castor oil, senna, bisacodyl
- Stool softeners—docusate, mineral oil, glycerin suppositories

## SECTION D
## *Musculoskeletal System Medications*

### 15.15 ANTI-INFLAMMATORIES

**Mechanisms and Sites of Action:**
- ASA—irreversibly inhibits cyclooxygenase, preventing prostaglandin and thromboxane formation
- NSAID—reversibly inhibits cyclooxygenase (COX) 1 and/or 2; COX 1 inhibition = gastritis and ulcer formation; COX 2 inhibition = dominant isoform during inflammation
- Corticosteroid—↓ inflammation by ↓ secretion of proinflammatory cytokines

**Primary Action(s) and Use(s):**
- ASA—1° indication—antipyretic, analgesic, anti-inflammatory, antiplatelet effects
- NSAID—1° indication—analgesic, anti-inflammatory
- Corticosteroid—1° indication—acute anti-inflammatory for short-term use

**Side Effects and Toxicity:**
- ASA—gastritis, ulcers, ↑ bleeding, Reye's syndrome; toxicity—tinnitus, fever, acute respiratory alkalosis → metabolic collapse and metabolic acidosis (overwhelms alkalosis)
- NSAID—↓ glomerular filtration rate with CHF, ↑ bleeding, GI upset, ulcers
- Corticosteroid—↑ risk for infection, peptic ulcers, GI hemorrhage, diabetes, HTN, psychosis, AVN, cataracts, severe osteoporosis, Cushing's syndrome, adrenal insufficiency

**Representative Drugs:**
- NSAIDs—ibuprofen, naproxen, celecoxib
- Corticosteroids—prednisone, methylprednisolone, dexamethasone

## 15.16A  AUTOIMMUNE DISEASES

**Mechanisms and Sites of Action:**
- Antimalarial—quinine derivatives, mechanism unknown
- Gold salts—mechanism is unknown
- Penicillamine—a metabolite of penicillin and analog of the amino acid cysteine; mechanism unknown
- Anti-TNF—key regulator of inflammation; 4 drugs used: (1) thalidomide inhibits secretion and peripheral effects of TNF; (2) pentoxifylline, phosphodiesterase inhibitor; (3) infliximab, neutralizes TNF; (4) etanercept, recombinant TNF receptor, neutralizes TNF in the bloodstream

**Primary Action(s) and Use(s):**
- Antimalarial—anti-inflammatory; 1° indication, SLE, RA, and other collagen vascular diseases
- Gold salts—retard the progression of bone and articular destruction; 1° indication = refractory RA
- Penicillamine—may retard the progression of bone and articular destruction; 1° indication = refractory RA
- Anti-TNF
    - Thalidomide—1° indication = leprosy, pyoderma gangrenosum, HIV-associated mucosal ulcers, multiple myeloma
    - Pentoxifylline—1° indication = PVD, improves survival in acute alcoholic hepatitis
    - Infliximab—1° indication = RA, Crohn's disease
    - Etanercept—1° indication = RA

*(continued)*

## 15.16B  AUTOIMMUNE DISEASES, Continued

**Side Effects and Toxicity:**
- Antimalarial—HA, pruritus, anorexia, malaise, urticaria, impaired hearing, confusion, psychosis, convulsions, blood dyscrasias, retinopathy, ototoxicity, myopathy, neuropathies, exfoliative dermatitis
- Penicillamine—blood dyscrasias, inhibition of wound healing, muscle and blood vessel damage, proteinuria, immune complex nephritis, skin and mucous membrane reactions, loss of taste perception, anorexia, N/V, may trigger a variety of autoimmune diseases, mammary hyperplasia, alopecia
- Anti-TNF
    - Thalidomide—severe birth defects
    - Pentoxifylline—dyspepsia, N/V, dizziness, HA, tremor, belching/bloating/flatus, angina/CP
    - Infliximab—transfusion reactions, delayed serum sickness, disseminated mycobacterial diseases with sudden sepsis
    - Etanercept—local injection reactions, sudden sepsis with disseminated mycobacterial infections

**Representative Drugs:**
- Antimalarial—chloroquine, hydroxychloroquine
- Penicillamine—Cuprimine
- Anti-TNF—thalidomide (Thalomid); pentoxifylline (Trental); infliximab (Remicade); etanercept (Enbrel)

# 15.17  MUSCLE RELAXANTS

**Mechanisms and Sites of Action:**
- Baclofen—GABA analog, works at the GABA-B receptors and serves a presynaptic inhibitory function
- Cyclobenzaprine—causes a reduction of tonic somatic motor activity, influencing both gamma and alpha motor systems
- Dantrolene—affects the contractile response of the skeletal muscle directly
- Diazepam—GABA-ergic enhancer

**Primary Action(s) and Use(s):**
- Baclofen—an active spasmolytic; 1° indication = ↓ spasticity
- Cyclobenzaprine—1° indication = muscle spasms associated with acute, painful musculoskeletal conditions
- Dantrolene—1° indication = spasticity from upper motor neuron disorders
- Diazepam—1° indication = skeletal muscle spasms, cerebral palsy, paraplegia

**Side Effects and Toxicity:**
- Baclofen—sedation, drowsiness, ↑ seizure threshold
- Cyclobenzaprine—drowsiness, dry mouth, fatigue, HA, dizziness
- Dantrolene—drowsiness, dizziness, weakness, general malaise, fatigue, diarrhea
- Diazepam—drowsiness, fatigue, ataxia, confusion, constipation, diplopia, HA, hypotension

**Representative Drugs:**
- Baclofen (Lioresal)
- Cyclobenzaprine (Flexeril)
- Dantrolene (Dantrium)
- Diazepam (Valium)

# SECTION E
## *Endocrine System Medications*

### 15.18A PITUITARY/HYPOTHALAMIC HORMONES

**Mechanisms and Sites of Action:**
- GnRH—suppresses FSH and LH release
- Somatotropin—(growth hormone) stimulates synthesis of somatomedins → longitudinal growth
- Somatostatin—inhibits somatotropin release from the pituitary and other hormones in the periphery
- Vasopressin (ADH)—acts on both $V_1$ and $V_2$ receptors:
  - $V_1$—vascular smooth muscle = vasoconstriction
  - $V_2$—renal collecting ducts = ↑ water resorption
- Oxytocin—stimulates milk secretion in lactating women and alters transmembrane ionic currents in myometrial smooth muscle cells to produce sustained uterine contraction

**Primary Action(s) and Use(s):**
- GnRH—1° indication = to suppress growth of endometriosis and prostate cancer
- Somatotropin—1° indication = to correct dwarfism, treat wasting in association with AIDS/CA
- Somatostatin—1° indication = Tx for variceal bleeding, carcinoid syndrome, vasoactive intestinal peptide-omas
- Vasopressin—1° indication = Tx of hypotension, pulseless ventricular tachycardia/fibrillation ($V_1$), central diabetes insipidus ($V_2$)
- Oxytocin—1° indication = to induce uterine contractions during labor

*(continued)*

## 15.18B PITUITARY/HYPOTHALAMIC HORMONES, Continued

**Side Effects and Toxicity:**
• GnRH—HA, ABD discomfort, flushing, bone pain, urinary tract symptoms, hot flashes
• Somatotropin—CREUTZFELDT–JAKOB DISEASE, slight ↑ risk of leukemia
• Somatostatin—ABD cramps, flatulence, diarrhea, bulky bowel movements, altered glucose tolerance
• Vasopressin—HA, nausea, abdominal cramps, allergic reactions; toxicity = hyponatremia
• Oxytocin—maternal death due to hypertensive crisis, uterine rupture, water intoxication and fetal deaths

**Representative Drugs:**
• GnRH—(gonadorelin, leuprolide)
• Somatotropin—(somatrem), human recombinant growth hormone
• Somatostatin—(Sandostatin)
• Vasopressin—(Pitressin tannate in oil), 8-arginine-vasopressin
• Oxytocin—(Pitocin, Syntocinon)

## 15.19A ADRENOCORTICOSTEROIDS

**Mechanisms and Sites of Action:**
• Zona glomerulosa—produces aldosterone naturally; agents = aldosterone, ACE inhibitors, mineralocorticoid analogs
• Zona fasciculata—produces corticosteroids naturally; agents = hydrocortisone, synthetic glucocorticoids
• Zona reticularis—produces testosterone naturally; agents = testosterone, DHEA, danazol

**Primary Action(s) and Use(s):**
• Aldosterone antagonists—1° indication = potassium-sparing diuretics
• ACE inhibitors—1° indication = antihypertensives
• Mineralocorticoid analogs—1° indication = Addison's disease
• Corticosteroids—1° indication = anti-inflammatory and antirejection
• Testosterone—1° indication = ↑ muscle mass in patients with CA, AIDS, or prolonged illness; hypogonadism, some autoimmune diseases (ITP)
   ○ Androgen inhibitors—each has own 1° indication—cyproterone = antihirsutism; flutamide = antiandrogen for prostate CA; finasteride = topically as hair-growth promoter, systemically for BPH

(continued)

## 15.19B ADRENOCORTICOSTEROIDS, Continued

**Side Effects and Toxicity:**
- Aldosterone antagonists—hypernatremia, hypokalemia, metabolic alkalosis, ↑ plasma volume, HTN
- ACE inhibitors—chronic cough, angioedema, hyperkalemia, ↑ creatinine
- Mineralocorticoid analogs—hypernatremia, hypokalemia, metabolic alkalosis, ↑ plasma volume, HTN
- Corticosteroids—iatrogenic Cushing's syndrome, muscle wasting, osteoporosis, diabetes, AVN, psychosis, impaired wound healing, thinning of the skin, peptic ulcers, cataracts, adrenal insufficiency
- Testosterone—masculinization, hirsutism

**Representative Drugs:**
- Aldosterone antagonists—spironolactone, amiloride, triamterene
- ACE inhibitors—captopril, enalapril, benazepril, lisinopril, fosinopril, ramipril
- Mineralocorticoid analogs—fludrocortisone, hydrocortisone
- Corticosteroids—prednisone, methylprednisolone, dexamethasone
- Testosterone—AndroGel, Striant mucoadhesive, Testim 1% Gel, Delatestryl
  - ○ Androgen inhibitors—cyproterone, flutamide, finasteride

## 15.20 THYROID HORMONES

**Note:** Regulated in part by an iodide pump in the thyroid

**Mechanisms and Sites of Action:** T4, T3, and rT3 are naturally occurring levoisomers; precise mechanism of action is controversial and there are multiple sites of action

**Primary Action(s) and Use(s):**
- T4—dominant circulating form, is converted to T3 in the periphery; 1° indication = hypothyroidism, replacement therapy after ablation or excision of gland for hyperthyroidism
- Antithyroid agents—agents that modify tissue response to thyroid hormones or destroy thyroid tissue; 1° indication = hyperthyroidism and thyroid storm

**Side Effects and Toxicity:**
- Thyroid preparations—resemble sympathetic nervous system overactivity (tachycardia, tremor, ↑ appetite)
- Antithyroid agents—maculopapular pruritic rash, fever, vasculitis, arthralgias, hepatitis, agranulocytosis

**Representative Drugs:**
- Thyroid preparations—levothyroxine, thyroglobulin (Synthroid, Levothroid)
- Antithyroid agents—iodide, iopanoic acid, methimazole, propylthiouracil

## 15.21A  HYPOGLYCEMIC AGENTS

**Mechanisms and Sites of Action:**
*Insulin:* Induces glucose uptake into tissues, shuts down gluconeogenesis and glycolysis
*Oral Hypoglycemics*
- Sulfonylureas—stimulate direct release of insulin from pancreatic beta islet cells
- Biguanides—upregulate insulin receptors and inhibits gluconeogenesis
- Thiazolidinediones—↑ tissue sensitivity to insulin
- Acarbose—inhibitor of α-glucosidase → interferes with carbohydrate digestion
- Meglitinide—stimulates insulin release from pancreas

**Primary Action(s) and Use(s):**
*Insulin:* 1° indication—Tx of diabetes, acute hyperkalemia
*Oral Hypoglycemics:* 1° indication—diabetes
- Sulfonylureas—DO NOT USE in sulfa-allergic patients
- Biguanides—1st line for obese diabetic patients; contraindicated in renal failure and CHF
- Thiazolidinediones, acarbose, meglitinide all indicated for diabetes without contraindications

*(continued)*

## 15.21B  HYPOGLYCEMIC AGENTS, Continued

**Side Effects and Toxicity:**
*Insulin:* Hypoglycemia, stimulation of anti-insulin antibodies, lipodystrophy at injection site
*Oral Hypoglycemics:* Hypoglycemia may occur with any:
- Sulfonylureas—weight gain, cholestatic jaundice, hepatitis, nausea, heartburn, allergic skin reactions
- Biguanides—lactic acidosis, URI, HA, back pain, fatigue, diarrhea, arthralgias, anemia
- Thiazolidinediones—hepatic failure, peripheral volume expansion, URI, HA, back pain, fatigue, sinusitis, diarrhea, anemia
- Acarbose—gas and ABD bloating, diarrhea
- Meglitinide—hypoglycemia, URI, HA, nausea, diarrhea, arthralgia

**Representative Drugs:**
*Insulin:* Regular, NPH
*Oral Hypoglycemics:*
- Sulfonylureas—glyburide, glipizide, glimepiride
- Biguanides—metformin
- Thiazolidinediones—pioglitazone, rosiglitazone
- Acarbose (Precose)
- Meglitinide—repaglinide

## 15.22A LIPID AGENTS

**Mechanisms and Sites of Action:**
- Binding resins—↑ excretion of bile acids → ↑ degradation of cholesterol to form more bile acids
- Niacin—inhibits triglyceride synthesis → ↓ VLDL → ↓ LDL
- Gemfibrozil—inhibits VLDL production and enhanced VLDL clearance = ↓ triglyceride > cholesterol, ↑ HDL
- HMG-CoA reductase inhibitors—limit the rate of cholesterol synthesis

**Primary Action(s) and Use(s):**
- Binding resins—1° indication = ↓ cholesterol with no effect on triglycerides
- Niacin—1° indication = cholesterol, ↑ HDL with slight ↓ triglycerides
- Gemfibrozil—1° indication = hypertriglyceridemia
- HMG-CoA reductase inhibitors—1° indication = 1st line therapy for hypercholesterolemia

*(continued)*

## 15.22B LIPID AGENTS, Continued

**Side Effects and Toxicity:**
- Binding resins—infection, HA, pain, flu syndrome, flatulence, constipation, diarrhea, nausea
- Niacin—cutaneous flushing, dizziness, syncope, tachycardia, palpitations, SOB, sweating, chills, edema
- Gemfibrozil—skin rash, GI and muscular symptoms, ↑ transaminases or alkaline phosphatase, potentiates action of anticoagulants
- HMG-CoA reductase inhibitors—diarrhea, constipation, ABD pain, flatulence, myalgias, HA, ↑ transaminases

**Representative Drugs:**
- Binding resins—(WelChol, colesevelam hydrochloride), colestipol, cholestyramine
- Niacin—(Advicor)
- Gemfibrozil—(Lopid)
- HMG-CoA reductase inhibitors—lovastatin, simvastatin, pravastatin, atorvastatin

## 15.23A  OSTEOPOROSIS AGENTS

**Note:** Calcium supplements recommended (> 1,200 mg/day) for all postmenopausal women as well as some type of weight bearing exercise to maintain bone health

**Mechanisms and Sites of Action:**
- Bisphosphonates—specific inhibitor of osteoclast-mediated bone resorption
- Calcitonin—mechanism not completely understood; causes a marked transient inhibition of the ongoing bone resorptive process
- Estrogens—bind to receptors in peripheral tissues

**Primary Action(s) and Use(s):**
- Bisphosphonates—coat hydroxyapatite with nonbiodegradable bisphosphonate shell; 1° indication—osteoporosis
- Calcitonin—↓ number of osteoclasts and an apparent ↓ in their resorptive activity; 1° indication = Paget's disease of bone, hypercalcemia, postmenopausal osteoporosis; also has analgesic properties in the Tx of osteoporotic compression fractures of the spine
- Estrogens—↓ vasomotor symptoms, vulvar and vaginal atrophy, and ↑ bone density; 1° indication = postmenopausal women

*(continued)*

## 15.23B  OSTEOPOROSIS AGENTS, Continued

**Side Effects and Toxicity:**
- Bisphosphonates—ABD pain, nausea, dyspepsia, constipation, diarrhea, musculoskeletal pain, HA
- Calcitonin—nausea, vomiting, facial flushing, skin rashes, poor appetite, ABD pain, edema of feet, possible allergic reactions including anaphylactic shock
- Estrogens—HA, pain, vaginal hemorrhage, URI, ↑ risk for endometrial CA, stroke, DVT, MI, breast CA, PE

**Representative Drugs:**
- Bisphosphonates—alendronate (Fosamax), pamidronate (Aredia)
- Calcitonin (Miacalcin)
- Estrogens (Premarin)

SECTION F
# *Neurologic System Medications*

## 15.24 NEUROGENIC AGENTS

**Mechanisms and Sites of Action:**
*Parkinsonian Agents:* Symptoms are due to imbalance between dopamine and acetylcholine
*Anesthetics*
- Local—stabilization of cell membrane, prevents depolarization of peripheral nerves
- General—affect cell membrane fluid dynamics

**Primary Action(s) and Use(s):**
*Parkinsonian Agents:* To ↑ ratio of dopamine to acetylcholine
*Anesthetics*
- Local
  - Topical = affects mucous membranes; infiltration = injection under skin
  - Regional blocks—injection of anesthetic medication into a specific site to cause anesthesia to a specific part of the body
- General—inhaled or IV, produces systemic analgesia

**Side Effects and Toxicity:**
*Parkinsonian Agents*
- Sinemet—nausea, psychosis, anxiety, arrhythmias, hyperkinesias/dyskinesias

- Amantadine—<u>LIVEDO</u> <u>RETICULARIS</u>, restlessness, hallucinations, urinary retention, dry mouth
*Anesthetics*
- Local—application site reactions, seizures, arrhythmias
- General—hypotension, respiratory depression, shock, death

**Representative Drugs:**
*Parkinsonian Agents*—levodopa-carbidopa (Sinemet), amantadine
*Anesthetics*
- Local—benzocaine, cocaine, chloroprocaine, lidocaine, bupivacaine
- General—propofol, fentanyl, ketamine, thiopental, diazepam

## 15.25  ANTISEIZURE AGENTS

**Mechanisms and Sites of Action:**
- Valproic acid—mechanism not established, related to ↑ GABA in brain
- Lamotrigine—mechanism unknown, possible effect on sodium channels
- Carbamazepine—↓ postsynaptic responses and blocks posttetanic potentiation
- Phenytoin—works in the motor cortex, possibly by ↓ membrane sodium gradient

**Primary Action(s) and Use(s):**
- Valproic acid—1° indication = 1st line in absence, tonic-clonic, simple, and complex partial seizures
- Lamotrigine—1° indication = 1st line in status epilepticus; 2nd line in absence, tonic-clonic, simple, and complex partial seizures
- Carbamazepine—1° indication = tonic-clonic, simple, and complex partial seizures
- Phenytoin—1° indication = simple and complex partial seizures and status epilepticus

**Side Effects and Toxicity:**
- Valproic acid—HA, N/V, ABD pain, diarrhea, somnolence, tremor, dizziness, diplopia, thrombocytopenia
- Lamotrigine—serious skin rash including Stevens-Johnson syndrome and toxic epidermal necrolysis, dizziness, ataxia, somnolence, HA, N/V
- Carbamazepine—dizziness, drowsiness, unsteadiness, N/V, aplastic anemia, agranulocytosis, severe skin reactions
- Phenytoin—nystagmus, ataxia, slurred speech, mental confusion, dizziness, insomnia, motor twitching, HA

**Representative Drugs:**
- Valproic acid (Depakene)
- Lamotrigine (Lamictal)
- Carbamazepine (Tegretol)
- Phenytoin (Phenytek)

# SECTION G
## *Psychiatric Medications*

### 15.26 ANTIPSYCHOTICS

**Mechanisms and Sites of Action:**
- Typical—block dopamine receptors (specifically D2)
- Atypical—less D2 blockage, more D4
- Mood stabilizers
  - Lithium—alters sodium transport in nerve and muscle cells, exact mechanism is unknown
  - Valproic acid and carbamazepine—used off-label, see antiseizure card (15.25) for specifics on these drugs

**Primary Action(s) and Use(s):**
- Typical—1° indication = hallucinations/delusions
- Atypical—1st line antipsychotic (due to ↓ side effects)
- Mood stabilizers
  - Lithium—1° indication = bipolar disorder
  - Valproic acid and carbamazepine—used off-label, used in the Tx of bipolar disorder

**Side Effects and Toxicity:**
- Typical—movement disorders, blurry vision, dry mouth, urinary retention, orthostatic hypotension, gynecomastia, amenorrhea, ↓ seizure threshold
- Atypical—dizziness, dry mouth, constipation, somnolence
- Mood stabilizers
  - Lithium—fine hand tremor, polyuria, thirst, nausea, diarrhea, vomiting, drowsiness, weakness, ataxia

**Representative Drugs:**
- Typical—haloperidol, chlorpromazine
- Atypical—risperidone, olanzapine
- Mood stabilizers—
  - Lithium (Eskalith)

## 15.27 ANTIDEPRESSANTS

**Mechanisms and Sites of Action:**
- SSRIs—inhibits CNS neuronal uptake of serotonin
- Tricyclics—inhibits reuptake of serotonin and norepinephrine at the presynaptic terminus
- MAOIs—irreversibly inhibit MAO isotypes A & B
- Bupropion—mechanism of action unknown; weak inhibitor of neuronal uptake of norepinephrine, serotonin, and dopamine

**Primary Action(s) and Use(s):**
- SSRIs—block uptake of serotonin into platelets—1° indications = depression, OCD, bulimia
- Tricyclics—1° indication = 2nd-line drugs for depression
- MAOIs—3rd-line agents for depression
- Bupropion—1° indication = depression, also used for smoking cessation

**Side Effects and Toxicity:**
- SSRIs—mild sedation, rare impotence; MUST avoid concurrent use with MAO inhibitors
- Tricyclics—sedation, blurry vision, dry mouth, urinary retention, severe orthostatic hypotension, TORSADE DE POINTES
- MAOIs—2 classic syndromes—SEROTONIN SYNDROME, HYPERTENSIVE CRISIS
- Bupropion—agitation, dry mouth, insomnia, HA, N/V, constipation, tremor

**Representative Drugs:**
- SSRIs—fluoxetine (Prozac), paroxetine (Paxil), sertraline (Zoloft)
- Tricyclics—amitriptyline (Elavil), desipramine (Norpramin)
- MAOIs—tranylcypromine (Parnate)
- Bupropion (Wellbutrin)

## 15.28 DEPRESSANTS

**Mechanisms and Sites of Action:**
- Benzodiazepines—anxiolytic properties similar, but different pharmacokinetics; divided into long, medium, and short half-life
- Barbiturates—bind to GABA receptors inhibiting neuronal signaling; divided into long, medium, and short half-life

**Primary Action(s) and Use(s):**
- Benzodiazepines—1° indications = anxiolytics, muscle relaxants, hypnotics, anesthetics
- Barbiturates—1° indication by class: long T1/2 = 2nd-line for seizures; medium T1/2 = sedative/hypnotics; short T1/2 = anesthetic agents

**Side Effects and Toxicity:**
- Benzodiazepines—confusion, impairment of driving skills, addiction/withdrawal, depression, tolerance; withdrawal effects = anxiety, insomnia, tremor, seizures
- Barbiturates—tolerance, addiction, fatal status epilepticus due to withdrawal, sedation

**Representative Drugs:**
- Benzodiazepines
  - Long half-life—diazepam, chlordiazepoxide
  - Medium half-life—alprazolam, lorazepam, temazepam
  - Short half-life—triazolam, midazolam, flumazenil
- Barbiturates
  - Long half-life—phenobarbital
  - Medium half-life—pentobarbital, secobarbital
  - Short half-life—thiopental, thiamylal

## 15.29A DRUGS OF ABUSE

**Opiates and Opioids**

*Heroin*

- "High"—rapid rush, short half-life (3–5 hr)
- Withdrawal begins 4–6 hr after last dose, peaks at 48 hr, subsides in 7–10 days
- Treatment
  - Addiction—methadone
  - OD—naloxone (Narcan) or naltrexone
  - Withdrawal—clonidine

**Stimulants**

*Cocaine*

- "High"—rapid rush, short half-life (1–2 hr)
- Withdrawal has 3 phases:
  1. The crash—irritability, confusion, dysphoria, +/– suicidal, insomnia, → sleeping 8–40 hr
  2. 2–10 weeks; sleep normalizes and mood improves, late → irritability and craving
  3. Baseline mood reestablished with episodic cravings
- Treatment
  - Addiction—psychotherapy and abstinence program
  - OD—usually fatal, if pt survives 3 hr or more, will usually recover; IV diazepam and propranolol

*Amphetamine*

- Very similar to cocaine except OD is rarely fatal and can be managed with IV haloperidol
- Withdrawal—paranoid psychosis (chronic use)

*Ecstasy (3,4-methylenedioxymethamphetamine, or MDMA):* Causes visual and other sensory hallucinations; ↑ perceptions; may cause a Parkinson-like state due to potent neurotoxicity

*(continued)*

## 15.29B DRUGS OF ABUSE, Continued

**Hallucinogens:**

*Lysergic Acid Diethylamide (LSD):* Causes sense inversion ("sees" sounds, "hears" colors, "smells" sights)

*Phencyclidine (PCP):* Causes psychosis, hallucinations, panic, violence, makes patient unaware of pain

*Mescaline:* Similar to LSD

Marijuana: Causes euphoria and relaxation, altered time perception, ↓ cognition, ↓ short-term memory, dose-dependent tachycardia and conjunctival injection, ↑ risk of bronchitis, asthma, and squamous cell metaplasia

# SECTION H
## *Hematologic System Medications*

### 15.30A ANTICOAGULANTS

**Mechanisms and Sites of Action:**
- Unfractionated heparin—inactivates thrombin
- Low-molecular-weight heparin—more specific at inhibiting factor X, more reliable bioavailability
- gpIIb/IIIa antagonists—reversibly inhibit platelet aggregation, based on cobra venom
- Lepirudin—direct inhibitor of thrombin; derivative of leech saliva
- Warfarin (Coumadin)—antagonizes vitamin K–dependent gamma carboxylation
- ASA—inhibits formation of platelet thromboxane
- Clopidogrel—inhibits ADP activation of platelet aggregation
- Drotrecogin alfa—inhibits intravascular coagulation

**Primary Action(s) and Use(s):**
- Unfractionated heparin—1° indication = prophylaxis for DVT, Tx of DVT and PE
- Low-molecular-weight heparin—1° indication = DVT prophylaxis and Tx
- gpIIb/IIIa antagonists—1° indication = as adjunct to heparin postangioplasty, MI, and unstable angina
- Lepirudin—1° indication = Tx of DVT in pts who cannot take heparin
- Warfarin—1° indication = outpatient therapy of DVT, atrial fibrillation
- ASA—1° indication = atrial fibrillation, MI, or CVA; 2nd-line oral anticoagulant
- Clopidogrel—1° indication = for pts who develop CVA while on ASA therapy
- Drotrecogin alfa—1° indication = sepsis

*(continued)*

## 15.30B  ANTICOAGULANTS, Continued

**Side Effects and Toxicity:**
- Unfractionated heparin—uncontrolled hemorrhage, heparin-induced thrombocytopenia
- Low-molecular-weight heparin—less bleeding and thrombocytopenia; not recommended for patients with bleeding diathesis due to longer half-life
- GP IIb/IIIa antagonists—severe hemorrhage
- Lepirudin—bleeding, abnormal LFTs, fever, pneumonia, allergic skin reactions
- Warfarin (Coumadin)—bleeding, "warfarin-induced skin necrosis" (rare)
- ASA—GI upset, bleeding, tinnitus
- Clopidogrel—TTP
- Drotrecogin alfa—bleeding

**Representative Drugs:**
- Unfractionated heparin—heparin
- Low-molecular-weight heparin (Lovenox)
- GP IIb/IIIa antagonists—eptifibatide, abciximab (ReoPro), tirofiban
- Lepirudin (Refludan)
- Warfarin (Coumadin)
- ASA
- Clopidogrel (Plavix)
- Drotrecogin alpha (Xigris)

## 15.31  THROMBOLYTICS

**Mechanisms and Sites of Action:**
- tPA—recombinant activator of plasmin, "fibrin-specific clot-buster"
- Streptokinase and urokinase—activate promolecule plasminogen

**Primary Action(s) and Use(s):**
- tPA—binds to fibrin in a thrombus and converts the entrapped plasminogen to plasmin, initiating local fibrinolysis; 1st-line for MI and ischemic stroke
- Streptokinase and urokinase—convert plasminogen to the enzyme plasmin; 1° indication—PE, MI

**Side Effects and Toxicity:** For all types—severe hemorrhage; hypersensitivity/anaphylactoid reactions

**Representative Drugs:**
- tPA—alteplase recombinant
- Streptokinase (Kabikinase, Streptase)
- Urokinase (Abbokinase)

## 15.32 HEMATOPOIETIC AGENTS

**Mechanisms and Sites of Action:**
- Recombinant erythropoietin—a glycoprotein that stimulates red blood cell production
- Filgrastim—a glycoprotein that stimulates the production of neutrophils
- Anagrelide—↓ platelet formation, exact mechanism is unknown

**Primary Action(s) and Use(s):**
- Recombinant erythropoietin—stimulates the division and differentiation of committed erythroid progenitors in bone marrow; 1° indication = anemia associated with CRF, HIV, or in CA patients on chemotherapy
- Filgrastim—1° indication = nonmyeloid malignancies, acute myeloid leukemia, CA patients receiving bone marrow transplants
- Anagrelide—1° indication = thrombocythemia of any cause

**Side Effects and Toxicity:**
- Recombinant erythropoietin—immunogenicity, fever, HTN, HA, fatigue, diarrhea, N/V
- Filgrastim—medullary bone pain
- Anagrelide—CHF, MI, cardiomyopathy, cardiomegaly, complete heart block, atrial fibrillation, CVA, pericarditis, pericardial effusion, pleural effusion, pulmonary infiltrates/fibrosis, pulmonary HTN, pancreatitis, gastric/duodenal ulcers, seizures

**Representative Drugs:**
- Recombinant erythropoietin (Epogen)
- Filgrastim (Neupogen)
- Anagrelide (Agrylin)

# SECTION I
## *Infectious Disease Medications*

### 15.33A ANTIBIOTICS: BACTERIAL CELL WALL INHIBITORS

**Penicillins:** Inhibit bacterial cell wall synthesis

- Resistance—β-lactamase production, altered PCN-binding proteins
- Toxicities—hypersensitivity reaction, leukopenia, induce autoimmune hemolytic anemia
- Bactericidal for actively dividing bacteria
- Coverage—simple PCN = *Strep.* agents and oral anaerobes
  - Aminopenicillins—↑ Gram-positive and anaerobic, + some community-acquired Gram-negative rods
  - Beta-lactamase inhibitors—↑ GP, GNR, and anaerobe coverage when added to aminopenicillins
  - Penicillinase-resistant penicillins—best *Staph.* coverage of all PCNs
  - Ureidopenicillins—broad-spectrum coverage, including nosocomial GNRs
- Rep Rx—penicillin, ampicillin, amoxicillin, methicillin, dicloxacillin

*(continued)*

## 15.33B ANTIBIOTICS: BACTERIAL CELL WALL INHIBITORS, Continued

**Cephalosporins:** Inhibit bacterial cell wall synthesis
- Resistance—beta-lactamase production, altered PCN-binding proteins
- Toxicities—15% cross-reactivity between PCN allergy and cephalosporin allergy
- Bactericidal for actively dividing bacteria
- Coverage
  - 1st generation—*Staph.* and *Strep.* is good, only OK community GNR
  - 2nd generation—worse *Staph.* coverage, better *Strep.,* GNR, and anaerobic
  - 3rd generation—↑ GNR coverage, GP coverage varies by drug; all penetrate CNS better than 1st or 2nd gen
- Rep Rx—cefazolin, cefuroxime, ceftriaxone

**Carbapenems:** Inhibit bacterial cell wall synthesis
- Resistance—altered PCN-binding proteins
- Toxicities—seizures
- Bactericidal for actively dividing bacteria
- Coverage—broadest spectrum coverage in any single agent
- Rep Rx—imipenem, meropenem

*(continued)*

## 15.33C ANTIBIOTICS: BACTERIAL CELL WALL INHIBITORS, Continued

**Monobactams:** Inhibit bacterial cell wall synthesis
- Resistance—altered PCN binding proteins
- Toxicities—minimal with no cross-reactivity to PCN
- Bactericidal for actively dividing bacteria
- Coverage—excellent GNR coverage
- Rep Rx—aztreonam

**Glycopeptide:** Inhibit bacterial cell wall synthesis
- Resistance—all GNs, some GPs
- Toxicities—renal toxicity; "red-man syndrome" (histamine-like reaction → skin turns red +/− respiratory compromise)
- Bacteriostatic
- Coverage—excellent for GPs, poor for GNs
- Rep Rx—vancomycin, bacitracin

## 15.34 ANTIBIOTICS: FOLATE ANTAGONISTS

**Trimethoprim:** Blocks dihydrofolate reductase—↓ production of folate
- Resistance—mutations in folate synthetic pathway and in targeted enzymes
- Toxicities—minimal
- Bacteriostatic
- Coverage—many GPCs and some GNRs

**Sulfonamides:** Inhibit folate synthesis
- Resistance—mutations in folate synthetic pathway and in targeted enzymes
- Toxicities—allergic reactions ranging from rash to anaphylaxis
- Bacteriostatic
- Coverage—many GPCs, some GNRs, and atypical organisms (*Actinomyces*)

**Trimethoprim/Sulfamethoxazole (Bactrim):** Synergistic block of the folate synthetic pathway
- Resistance—mutations in folate synthetic pathway and in targeted enzymes
- Toxicities—allergic reactions common
- Bactericidal
- Coverage—GPCs, GNRs, and atypicals well; ↑ concentrations in kidney, urine, and prostate = ideal for uncomplicated UTIs, kidney infections, and GU infections

## 15.35A ANTIBIOTICS: PROTEIN SYNTHESIS INHIBITORS

**Aminoglycosides:** Blocks protein synthesis initiation
- Resistance—altered uptake of drug; bacterial enzymes modify drugs' structures, inactivating them; mutations in bacterial ribosomes blocks drug's ability to bind to target; anaerobes are intrinsically resistant
- Toxicities—renal tubular damage and ototoxicity
- Bactericidal
- Coverage—1st line for GNs, excellent for nosocomial GNRs; for GPCs, must synergize with cell wall inhibitors
- Rep Rx—streptomycin, gentamicin, neomycin, tobramycin

**Tetracyclines:** Inhibit protein synthesis
- Resistance—due to ↓ uptake
- Toxicities—discoloration of teeth in children, photosensitize skin; sunburns
- Bacteriostatic
- Coverage—fairly broad spectrum, most useful for intracellular, atypical bacteria
- Absorption—in the gut, inhibited by antacids
- Rep Rx—doxycycline, demeclocycline, tetracycline

*(continued)*

## 15.35B ANTIBIOTICS: PROTEIN SYNTHESIS INHIBITORS, Continued

**Chloramphenicol:** Inhibits formation of peptide bond
- Resistance—acetylation of the drug, or ↓ drug uptake
- Toxicities—aplastic anemia, gray-baby syndrome (cyanosis and shock)
- Bacteriostatic
- Coverage—very broad spectrum (GPs, GNRs, atypical/intracellular and many anaerobes)

**Macrolides:** Interfere with protein synthesis
- Resistance—due to ↓ cell uptake, enzymatic inactivation, or mutations
- Toxicities—GI upset, N/V, diarrhea, drug interactions → torsade de pointes
- Bacteriostatic
- Coverage
  - 1st generation—*Strep. and atypicals*
  - 2nd generation—excellent *Strep.* and atypical, minimal GNs
- Rep Rx—erythromycin, clarithromycin, azithromycin

*(continued)*

## 15.35C ANTIBIOTICS: PROTEIN SYNTHESIS INHIBITORS, Continued

**Lincosamide:** Blocks formation of peptide bond
- Resistance—2° to mutations
- Toxicities—*C. difficile* infection 2° to killing GI flora
- Bactericidal for GPC, bacteriostatic for anaerobes
- Coverage—GPC, excellent coverage for anaerobes
- Rep Rx—clindamycin

**Streptogramins:** Inhibit protein synthesis
- Resistance—GN and *Enterococcus faecalis*
- Toxicities—severe thrombophlebitis
- Bacteriostatic
- Coverage—most GPs (including VREs), and MRSAs
- Rep Rx—quinupristin, dalfopristin

**Oxazolidinone:** Stops protein synthesis before it starts
- Resistance—rare *Enterococcus*
- Toxicities—anemia and thrombocytopenia
- Bacteriostatic
- Coverage—all GPCs
- Rep Rx—linezolid

## 15.36 ANTIBIOTICS: NUCLEIC ACID INHIBITORS

**Fluoroquinolones:** Block activity of DNA gyrase
- Resistance—due to mutations
- Toxicities—may cause bone or joint disease in children, including tendon rupture
- Bactericidal
- Coverage—excellent GNs, atypical, intracellular, and nosocomial GNRs; newer agents have GP coverage
- Rep Rx—ciprofloxacin, levofloxacin, gatifloxacin, ofloxacin

**Rifamycins:** Inhibit RNA polymerase
- Resistance—develops during monotherapy
- Toxicities—turns body secretions orange/red
- Bactericidal
- Coverage—1st line as combination therapy for TB, endocarditis, osteomyelitis, meningitis
- Rep Rx—rifampin, rifabutin

## 15.37A ANTIBIOTICS: MISCELLANEOUS AGENTS

**Metronidazole:** Poisons anaerobic metabolism
- Resistance—due to slow drug uptake
- Toxicities—has a disulfiram-like effect with alcohol, causes metallic aftertaste
- Bactericidal
- Coverage—most effective agent for bowel anaerobes
- Rep Rx—Metronidazole

**Isoniazid:** Inhibits mycolic acid synthesis
- Resistance—develops during monotherapy if organism burden is high enough
- Toxicities—risk of fulminant hepatic toxicity, also ↓ B6
- Bactericidal
- Coverage—extremely effective for TB and other mycobacteria
- Rep Rx—isoniazid

**Ethambutol:** Mechanism unknown
- Resistance—unusual with combination therapy, common with monotherapy
- Toxicities—optic nerve and retinal toxicity
- Bactericidal
- Coverage—part of a 4-drug therapy for TB (rifampin, isoniazid, pyrazinamide, ethambutol; the RIPE drugs)

*(continued)*

## 15.37B ANTIBIOTICS: MISCELLANEOUS AGENTS, Continued

**Pyrazinamide:** Mechanism unclear
- Resistance—unusual during combination therapy
- Toxicities—hepatoxicity
- Bactericidal
- Coverage—one of the "RIPE" drugs for TB

**Dapsone:** Mechanism unclear
- Resistance—will emerge with monotherapy in patients with large organism burden
- Toxicities—hemolysis can occur, also methemoglobinemia and GI upset
- Bactericidal
- Coverage—1st line for leprosy; 2nd line for *Pneumocystis carinii*

## 15.38A ANTIVIRALS

**Acyclovir:** Inhibits DNA polymerase and acts as a DNA chain terminator
- Resistance—becoming a problem
- Toxicities—CNS, renal failure
- Coverage—1st line for herpes simplex and varicella zoster, does not cover cytomegalovirus

**Valacyclovir:** Similar to acyclovir but has a longer half-life

**Ganciclovir:** Inhibits viral DNA polymerase, does not act as a chain terminator
- Resistance—less common than with acyclovir
- Toxicities—neutropenia
- Coverage—1st line for CMV

**Penciclovir:** Inhibits viral DNA polymerase; does not lead to DNA chain termination
- Resistance—cross-resistance with acyclovir
- Toxicities—mild
- Coverage—HSV-1, HSV-2, VZV

**Cidofovir:** Activated by cellular phosphorylases, not viral phosphorylases
- Resistance—unusual
- Toxicities—nephrotoxicity and neutropenia
- Coverage—broad-spectrum coverage, HSV-1 HSV-2, VZV, CMV, EBV

*(continued)*

## 15.38B  ANTIVIRALS, Continued

**Foscarnet:** Directly inhibits viral DNA polymerase or reverse transcriptase
- Resistance—rare
- Toxicities—nephrotoxicity
- Coverage—covers ganciclovir-resistant CMV, VZV, HSV, and HIV

**Idoxuridine:** Inhibits DNA replication
- Resistance—occasional
- Toxicities—topical allergic/irritant reactions
- Coverage—used topically only for HSV keratitis

**Amantadine:** Inhibits viral uncoating after entry into cell
- Resistance—not a major clinical problem
- Toxicities—seizures and arrhythmias
- Coverage—shortens duration of influenza A virus

**Rimantadine:** Similar to amantadine

**Lamivudine (3TC):** Inhibits reverse transcriptase of both hepatitis B virus and HIV
- Resistance—develops during monotherapy
- Toxicities—hepatic failure
- Coverage—chronic HBV and in combination therapy for HIV

*(continued)*

## 15.38C  ANTIVIRALS, Continued

**Ribavirin:** Inhibits a number of viral enzymes, inhibiting RNA/DNA synthesis
- Resistance—not clinically seen
- Toxicities—hemolysis and bone marrow suppression
- Coverage—broad spectrum, 1st line for RSV, in combo with interferon-α for chronic hepatitis C

**Zanamivir:** Inhibits the neuraminidase enzyme of influenza A and B
- Resistance—not a clinical problem
- Toxicities—mild bronchospasm (an inhaled drug)
- Coverage—1st line for prophylaxis of influenza in close contacts, shortens duration of influenza when started early

**Oseltamivir:** Inhibits the neuraminidase enzyme of influenza A and B
- Resistance—not a clinical problem
- Toxicities—mild GI upset (orally administered)
- Coverage—1st line for prophylaxis of influenza in close contacts, shortens duration of influenza when started early

**Interferon-α:** Stimulates cells to resist viral infection by multiple mechanisms
- Resistance—none
- Toxicities—severe flu-like symptoms, severe depression
- Coverage—chronic HBV and with ribavirin for chronic HCV

## 15.39A  ANTIFUNGALS

**Polyenes:** Bind to ergosterol in the fungal cell membrane
- Resistance—unusual
- Toxicities—severe rigors and malaise, also cause dose-dependent renal insufficiency and renal tubular acidosis with potassium and magnesium wasting
- Bactericidal
- Coverage—broadest spectrum antifungal agents available; 1st line for serious infections

**Azoles:** Inhibit ergosterol synthesis by disrupting the cytochrome P450 pathway
- Resistance—an increasingly common problem
- Toxicities—GI intolerance, cholestasis, hepatitis
- Bacteriostatic
- Coverage—cover yeast very well, but must be used with caution in neutropenic patients

**5-flucytosine (5FC):** Inhibits DNA synthesis in fungal cells
- Resistance—expected in monotherapy; always combine with 2nd agent
- Toxicities—bone marrow suppression
- Bactericidal
- Coverage—1st line for cryptococcal meningitis

*(continued)*

## 15.39B  ANTIFUNGALS, Continued

**Terbinafine:** Inhibits ergosterol synthesis by interfering with precursor assembly
- Resistance—not a clinical problem
- Toxicities—severe hepatitis
- Bacteriostatic
- Coverage—onychomycosis

**Griseofulvin:** Mechanism unclear
- Resistance—develops with prolonged therapy
- Toxicities—severe hepatitis, GI upset
- Bacteriostatic
- Coverage—onychomycosis

**Echinocandins:** Inhibit a key enzyme in the synthesis of fungal cell walls
- Resistance—unclear
- Toxicities—unclear
- Bactericidal
- Coverage—*Aspergillus*
- Rep Rx—caspofungin

## 15.40A ANTIPARASITICS

**Metronidazole:** Mechanism unknown
- Toxicities—has a disulfiram-like effect with alcohol, causes a metallic aftertaste
- Coverage—GI and vaginal protozoa, especially *Entamoeba, Giardia,* and *Trichomonas*

**Iodoquinol:** Mechanism unknown
- Toxicities—iodine-related skin irritation and thyroid dysfunction
- Coverage—used in combination with metronidazole to treat *Entamoeba*

**Quinine:** Mechanism unknown
- Toxicities—hemolysis and retinal toxicity
- Coverage—*Plasmodium* spp.

*(continued)*

## 15.40B ANTIPARASITICS, Continued

**Folate Antagonists:** Blocks folate synthesis
- Toxicities—allergic reactions to sulfa moieties, hemolysis
- Coverage—1st line for *Toxoplasma,* in combination with sulfadiazine for *Plasmodium* and *Pneumocystis*

**Pentamidine:** Mechanism unknown
- Toxicities—numerous: allergic reactions, pancreatitis, hypoglycemia, renal failure
- Coverage—2nd line in aerosolized form for *Pneumocystis*

**Pyrantel Pamoate:** Acts as a depolarizing neuromuscular blocking agent in helminths
- Toxicities—minimal
- Coverage—for intestinal nematodes, principally *Enterobius*

**Niclosamide:** Inhibits oxidative phosphorylation in worms
- Toxicities—minimal toxicities
- Coverage—all tapeworms except *Taenia solium*

# Abbreviations

| | | | |
|---|---|---|---|
| +/− | with or without | BMI | body mass index |
| < | less than | BP | blood pressure |
| = | equal to | BPH | benign prostatic hypertrophy |
| > | greater than | bpm | beats per minute |
| 1° | primary | BS | bowel sounds |
| 2° | secondary | BSA | body surface area |
| AAA | abdominal aortic aneurysm | C&S | culture and sensitivity |
| ABD | abdomen/abdominal | CA | cancer |
| ABG | arterial blood gases | CABG | coronary artery bypass grafting |
| AC | acromioclavicular | CAD | coronary artery disease |
| ACE | angiotensin converting enzyme | CAP | community-acquired pneumonia |
| ACL | anterior cruciate ligament | CBC | complete blood cell count |
| ADH | antidiuretic hormone | CCU | coronary care unit |
| ADLs | activities of daily living | CF | cystic fibrosis |
| AFP | alpha-fetoprotein | CFL | calcaneofibular ligament |
| ALL | acute lymphoblastic leukemia | CHF | congestive heart failure |
| ALOC | altered level of consciousness | CMV | cytomegalovirus |
| AM | morning | CN | cranial nerve |
| AMI | acute myocardial infarction | CNS | central nervous system |
| AML | acute myelogenous leukemia | CO | cardiac output |
| ANA | antinuclear antibodies | COA | coarctation of the aorta |
| AP | anteroposterior | COPD | chronic obstructive pulmonary disease |
| APL | abductor pollicis longus | CP | chest pain |
| AR | atrial regurgitation | CPAP | continuous positive airway pressure |
| ARDS | adult respiratory distress syndrome | CRP | C-reactive protein |
| AROM | active range of motion | CSF | cerebrospinal spinal fluid |
| ASA | acetylsalicylic acid (aspirin) | CT | computed tomography |
| ASD | atrial septal defect | CTS | carpal tunnel syndrome |
| ATFL | anterior talofibular ligament | CVA | cerebrovascular accident |
| ATN | acute tubular necrosis | Cx | cultures |
| AV | atrioventricular | CXR | chest x-ray |
| AVM | atrioventricular malformation | db | decibel |
| AVN | avascular necrosis | D&C | dilation and curettage |
| B/L | bilateral | DC | discontinue (stop) |
| BBB | bundle branch block | DIC | disseminated intravascular coagulation |
| BE | barium enema | DIP | distal interphalangeal |
| bid | two times per day | DJD | degenerative joint disease |
| BM | bowel movement | DKA | diabetic ketoacidosis |

| | | | |
|---|---|---|---|
| DM | diabetes mellitus | IDDM | insulin-dependent diabetes mellitus |
| DRE | digital rectal exam | IM | intramuscular |
| DTRs | deep tendon reflexes | IR | internal rotation |
| DUB | dysfunctional uterine bleeding | ITP | idiopathic thrombocytopenic purpura |
| DVT | deep venous thrombosis | IUD | intrauterine device |
| Dx | diagnosis | IV | intravenous |
| Dz | disease | IVC | intravenous contrast |
| EBV | Epstein-Barr virus | IVDA | intravenous drug abuse |
| ECG | electrocardiogram | IVIG | intravenous immunoglobulin |
| echo | echocardiogram | JVD | jugular vein distention |
| ECRB | extensor carpi radialis brevis | L | left |
| ECT | electroconvulsive therapy | LAD | left axis deviation |
| ED | emergency department | LAH | left atrial hypertrophy |
| EEG | electroencephalogram | LE | lower extremity |
| EMG | electromyogram | LES | lower esophageal sphincter |
| EPB | extensor pollicis brevis | LFT | liver function tests |
| ER | external rotation | LLQ | left lower quadrant |
| ERCP | endoscopic retrograde cholangiopancreatography | LOC | level of consciousness |
| | | LP | lumbar puncture |
| ESR | erythrocyte sedimentation rate | LUQ | left upper quadrant |
| ESRD | end-stage renal disease | LV | left ventricular |
| ETOH | ethyl alcohol | LVH | left ventricular hypertrophy |
| F | female | M | male |
| FB | foreign body | MAOIs | monoamine oxidase inhibitors |
| FCR | flexor carpi radialis | MCP | metacarpophalangeal |
| $FEV_1$ | forced expiratory volume | MI | myocardial infarction |
| FFP | fresh frozen plasma | MR | mitral regurgitation |
| $FiO_2$ | fractional inspiration of oxygen | ms | mental status |
| FNA | fine needle aspirate | MS | mitral stenosis |
| FVC | forced ventilatory capacity | M.S. | multiple sclerosis |
| Fx | fractured | MSO4 | morphine sulfate |
| GERD | gastroesophageal reflux disease | MUA | manipulation under anesthesia |
| GFR | glomerular filtration rate | MVP | mitral valve prolapse |
| GI | gastrointestinal | N/V | nausea/vomiting |
| GnRH | gonadotropin-releasing hormone | NG | nasogastric |
| GPR | Gram-positive rod | NGT | nasogastric tube |
| GU | genitourinary | NIDDM | non-insulin-dependent diabetes mellitus |
| H&P | history and physical | NPO | nothing by mouth |
| HA | headache | NSAIDs | nonsteroidal anti-inflammatory drug |
| HAP | hospital-acquired pneumonia | NSR | normal sinus rhythm |
| HAV | hepatitis A virus | NTG | nitroglycerin |
| HBV | hepatitis B virus | NWB | non weight bearing |
| HCV | hepatitis C virus | $O_2$ | oxygen |
| HEV | hepatitis E virus | O&P | ova and parasites |
| HF | heart failure | OA | osteoarthritis |
| HIV | human immunodeficiency virus | OCD | obsessive compulsive disorder |
| HPV | human papillomavirus | OCP | oral contraceptive pills |
| HRT | hormone replacement therapy | OD | overdose |
| HSV | herpes simplex virus | OM | otitis media |
| HTN | hypertension | OR | operating room |
| HUS | hemolytic-uremic syndrome | ORIF | open reduction and internal fixation |
| I&D | incision and drainage (or irrigation and débridement) | OT | occupational therapy |
| | | OTC | over the counter |
| IBD | inflammatory bowel disease | P.T. | pronator teres |
| IBS | irritable bowel syndrome | P/E | physical exam |
| IC | intercostal | PCN | penicillin |
| ICS | intercostal space | $PCO_2$ | partial pressure of carbon dioxide |
| ID | identify | PDA | patent ductus arteriosus |

| | | | | |
|---|---|---|---|---|
| PE | pulmonary embolus | | SA | sinoatrial |
| PEEP | positive end-expiratory pressure | | SB | sternal border |
| PFT | pulmonary function test | | SBFT | small bowel follow-through |
| phpf | per high-power field | | SCD | sequential compression device |
| PID | pelvic inflammatory disease | | SI | sacroiliac |
| PIP | proximal interphalangeal | | SLE | systemic lupus erythematosus |
| PKD | polycystic kidney disease | | SOB | shortness of breath |
| PLL | posterior longitudinal ligament | | sp/st | sprain/strain |
| PM | evening | | SQ | subcutaneous |
| PMI | point of maximum impulse | | SSRIs | selective serotonin reuptake inhibitors |
| PMS | premenstrual syndrome | | STD | sexually transmitted disease |
| PND | paroxysmal nocturnal dyspnea | | SVR | systemic vascular resistance |
| PO | per os (by mouth) | | SVT | supraventricular tachycardia |
| PPD | purified protein derivative | | TB | tuberculosis |
| PPI | proton pump inhibitor | | TBSA | total body surface area |
| PRN | pro re nata (as needed) | | TFT | thyroid function test |
| PROM | passive range of motion | | TIA | transient ischemic attack |
| PS | pulmonary stenosis | | tid | ter in die (three times a day) |
| pt | patient | | TLC | total lung capacity |
| PT | physical therapy | | TM | tympanic membrane |
| PTCA | percutaneous transluminal coronary angioplasty (+/− stent) | | TNF | tumor necrosis factor |
| | | | TOF | tetralogy of Fallot |
| PTH | parathyroid hormone | | TPN | total parenteral nutrition |
| PVCs | premature ventricular contractions | | TR | tricuspid regurgitation |
| PVD | peripheral vascular disease | | TS | tricuspid stenosis |
| q | every | | TSH | thyroid-stimulating hormone |
| qid | quater in die (four times a day) | | TTP | tenderness to palpation |
| R | right | | TURP | transurethral resection of the prostate |
| RA | rheumatoid arthritis | | TX | treatment |
| RAD | right axis deviation | | U | units |
| RBCs | red blood cells | | UA | urinalysis |
| RF | renal failure | | UGI | upper gastrointestinal |
| RFT | renal function test | | URI | upper respiratory infection |
| RICE | rest, ice, compression, elevation | | US | ultrasound |
| RLQ | right lower quadrant | | UTI | urinary tract infection |
| ROM | range of motion | | VDRL | Venereal Disease Research Laboratory |
| RPR | rapid plasma reagin | | V/Q | ventilation/perfusion |
| RSD | reflex sympathetic dystrophy | | VS | vital signs |
| rtPA | recombinant tissue plasminogen activator | | VSD | ventricular septal defect |
| RUQ | right upper quadrant | | VWF | von Willebrand factor |
| RV | right ventricle | | WBCs | white blood cells |
| R.V. | residual volume | | X | times |
| RVH | right ventricular hypertrophy | | XR | x-ray |
| $S_3$ | third heart sound | | XRT | x-ray therapy (radiation treatment) |
| $S_4$ | fourth heart sound | | Y/O | years old |
| S/S | signs/symptoms | | Z-E syndrome | Zollinger-Ellison syndrome |

# Terminology Links

The following descriptions of specific entities and constellations of symptoms define the terms identified on the review cards in small capital letters. They are organized here first by chapter and then in alphabetical order by review card number/title.

| Review Card Number/Title | Terminology Links |
| --- | --- |
| **Chapter 1: Cardiovascular System** | |
| 1.3: Aortic Aneurysm | **superior vena cava syndrome**—dilation of collateral veins of the upper chest and neck; edema and plethora of the face, neck, and upper torso and breasts; suffusion and edema of the conjunctiva; breathlessness in the supine position; and CNS symptoms (HA, visual disturbances, ALOC) |
| 1.4: Atrioventricular (AV) Heart Blocks | **Stokes-Adams attack**—altered level of consciousness due to decreased cerebral blood flow secondary to transient decreased cardiac output. May be light-headed, dizzy, or progress to unconsciousness with possible convulsions |
| 1.5: Bacterial Endocarditis | **Janeway lesions**—painless hemorrhagic plaques on palms and soles |
| | **Osler's nodes**—painful erythematous subcutaneous nodular lesions on the tips of the digits |
| | **Roth's spots**—pale retinal round or oval lesions surrounded by hemorrhage |
| 1.9A: Cardiomyopathy | **Pulsus bisferiens**—a notch or dip in midsystole, results in a "double beating" sensation on palpation |
| 1.14: Congenital Heart Defects: Tetralogy of Fallot | **"Tet spells"**—periodic episodic cyanosis and agitation caused by an increase in RV outflow tract resistance, leading to an increase in the R to L shunt |
| 1.17: Coronary Artery Disease | **Levine's sign**—clenched fist over the chest |
| 1.18: Deep Venous Thrombosis | **Homans' sign**—pain in calf with forced dorsiflexion of ankle |
| | **Trousseau's sign**—migratory thrombophlebitis—venous thromboses that spontaneously appear, disappear, and reappear elsewhere (usually due to malignancy) |
| | **Virchow's triad**—stasis or immobility (post-op, long car or plane ride); hypercoagulability (CA, nephritic syndrome, pregnancy, OCP, obesity); endothelial trauma (infection, IV catheters, fractures) |
| 1.20: Dysrhythmias: Bradydysrhythmias, Specific Types | **sick sinus syndrome**—sinus node dysfunction with symptomatic bradycardia |
| 1.22B: Dysrhythmias: Tachydysrhythmias, Specific Types, Continued | **torsade de pointes**—ventricular tachycardia in which QRS appear to be "twisting"; usually secondary to electrolyte imbalance, severe cardiomyopathies or congenitally long-QT syndrome |

| Review Card Number/Title | Terminology Links |
|---|---|
| 1.25: Hypertension | **Keith-Wagner-Barker classification**—(Card 5.14) |
| 1.26: Hypertension, Specific Types | **cor pulmonale**—hypertrophy or failure of right ventricle resulting from disorders of the lungs, pulmonary vessels, or chest wall |
| | **Raynaud's phenomenon**—intermittent episodes in which digits go from pallor to cyanosis then redness. Episodes may be triggered by exposure to cold or emotional stresses and may be accompanied by numbness, tingling, and/or burning. |
| 1.28: Myocardial Infarction | **Dressler's syndrome**—an autoimmune pleuropericarditis associated with fever and elevated ESR; usually presents weeks after initial infarct |
| 1.30: Pericardial Disorders | **Beck's triad**—tachycardia, tachypnea, and pulsus paradoxus–classic diagnostic presentation of cardiac tamponade |
| | **electrical alternans**—alternating low-voltage and normal voltage complexes on ECG |
| | **Ewart's sign**—bronchial breath sounds audible in the left upper lobe |
| | **Kussmaul's sign**—neck vein distention on inspiration |
| | **pulsus paradoxus**—accentuation of the normal inspiratory decline in systemic systolic BP |
| 1.32: Peripheral Vascular Disease | **ankle brachial index (ABI)**—normally systolic BP in legs is higher than in arms, ABI is greater than 1.0. Values < 0.9 predict PVD, those < 0.5 indicate severe ischemia and are prognostic for healing potential (lack of) |
| | **intermittent claudication**—lower extremity pain or tightness and cramping with exercise; symptoms occur at a relatively constant level of exertion and disappear with rest |
| | **Leriche's syndrome**—aortoiliac disease (symptoms in buttock, hip, and thigh) with associated impotence |
| 1.34: Rheumatic Heart Disease | **erythema marginatum**—a serpiginous, flat, painless rash |
| | **Sydenham's chorea**—rapid, purposeless movements that occur only while awake; "bag of worms" of tongue upon protrusion |
| 1.37: Valvular Diseases: Aortic Regurgitation | **Corrigan's pulse**—sharp, rapid carotid upstroke with subsequent collapse |
| | **de Musset's sign**—systolic head bobbing |
| | **Duroziez's murmur**—to-and-fro bruit at the femoral artery |
| | **Hill's sign**—systolic BP in leg > 20 mmHg higher than in arm |
| | **Muller's sign**—systolic bobbing of the uvula |
| | **Quincke's pulse**—nail bed capillary pulsation upon gentle nail pressure |
| | **Traube's sign**—pistol-shot sounds over the radial or femoral artery |
| 1.42: Valvular Diseases: Tricuspid Regurgitation | **Carvallo's sign**—increased intensity of the pansystolic murmur with inspiration |

## Chapter 2: Pulmonary System

| | |
|---|---|
| 2.3: Asthma | **pulsus paradoxus**—accentuation of the normal inspiratory decline in systemic systolic BP |
| | **status asthmaticus**—persistent, severe attack, refractory to treatment; may lead to respiratory failure and death |
| 2.5: Bronchiectasis | **"signet ring" bronchioles**—a dilated bronchus (the ring) with a visible associated pulmonary artery (the stone) |
| | **"tram tracks"**—dilated airways parallel to each other due to collapse of intervening alveoli |
| 2.6: Bronchiolitis | **BOOP—bronchiolitis obliterans organizing pneumonia;** causes obstruction of bronchioles by granulation and fibrous tissue |
| 2.15: Pneumonia | **egophony**—a nasal sound heard in auscultation of the chest when the subject speaks in a normal tone; indicates pleural effusion |
| 2.17: Pneumothorax | **tactile fremitus**—vibration or thrill felt while the patient is speaking and the hand is held against the chest |
| 2.18: Pulmonary Embolism | **Homans' sign**—pain in the calf when the toe is passively dorsiflexed; an early sign in DVT of deep veins of the calf |

| Review Card Number/Title | Terminology Links |
|---|---|
| **Chapter 3: Gastrointestinal System and Nutrition** ||
| 3.3: Alcoholic Liver Disease | **cirrhosis** (Card 3.6) |
| | **hepatitis** (Cards 3.18 to 3.20B) |
| | **acute pancreatitis** (Card 14.12) |
| | **chronic pancreatitis** (Card 3.32) |
| 3.6: Cirrhosis | **caput medusa**—plexus of dilated veins around the umbilicus; indicates portal vein obstruction |
| 3.9: Crohn's Disease | **skip lesions**—alternating areas of disease with normal mucosa |
| | **"string sign"**—thin string of contrast; indicates lumen of ileum compressed from edematous bowel wall |
| 3.31: Pancreatic Carcinoma | **Courvoisier's sign**—palpable, enlarged gallbladder |
| 3.34: Sclerosing Cholangitis, Primary | **Crohn's disease** (Card 3.9) |
| | **ulcerative colitis** (Card 3.37) |
| **Chapter 4: Musculoskeletal System** ||
| 4.2: Ankle Fracture | **Maisonneuve's fracture**—fracture of medial malleolus with complete disruption of the syndesmosis and proximal fibular shaft fracture |
| 4.3: Ankle Sprain | **Ottawa ankle rules**—indicates need for x-rays if any of the following are present: (1) TTP at posterior tip of lateral malleolus; (2) TTP at posterior tip of medial malleolus; (3) inability to bear weight at the time of injury or exam |
| | **talar tilt test**—plantarflexed ankle, invert talus from stabilized tibia; + test = ↑ laxity from uninjured side |
| 4.5: Anterior Cruciate Ligament (ACL) Injury | **Lachman's test**—with knee at 30° flexion, examiner stabilizes the femur and anteriorly translates tibia on the stabilized femur; + test shows ↑ anterior translation from uninjured side |
| | **pivot shift test**—examiner grasps foot and internally rotates tibia with knee in extension → anteriorly subluxed the anterolateral portion of the tibia → flex knee slowly → tibia will reduce 2° to ITB tightening and is + exam |
| | **Segond fracture**—avulsion fracture of the proximal lateral tibial cortex; associated with ACL +/− MCL injury |
| 4.11: Cubital Tunnel Syndrome | **Froment's sign**—with pinching of paper between thumb and index finger, the thumb IP joint flexes to substitute for weak adductor pollicis muscles |
| 4.12: de Quervain's Tenosynovitis | **Finkelstein's test**—ulnar deviation of the wrist with the thumb flexed into the palm of the hand; pain over the 1st dorsal compartment of the wrist is + test |
| 4.13: Dysplasia of the Hip, Developmental | **Barlow test**—direct pressure on longitudinal axis of the femur as flexed hip is moved from adduction to abduction, positive = subluxation of femoral head out of acetabulum |
| | **Galeazzi's sign**—asymmetrical knee heights with patient supine and hips and knees flexed to 90° |
| | **Ortolani test**—gentle abduction of flexed hip with slight upward pressure on posterior aspect of hip, positive = click as femoral head reduces |
| | **Trendelenburg gait**—"waddling" gait 2° to patient lurching toward affected hip, placing center of gravity directly over the hip to compensate for weak gluteus medius muscle |
| 4.14: Epicondylitis, Lateral | **"coffee cup test"**—pain with grasping or pinching with the wrist in extension |
| 4.18: Gout | **Martel's sign**—"punched out" lytic areas with overhanging bony edges |
| | **podagra**—first MTP joint pain, swelling, erythema |
| 4.20: Hand Infections: Flexor Tenosynovitis | **Kanavel's signs**—pain on passive extension, digit held in flexed position, exquisite tenderness along flexor tendon sheath, fusiform swelling |

| Review Card Number/Title | Terminology Links |
|---|---|
| 4.23A: Low Back Pain | **radiculopathy**—radiation of pain or numbness to extremity due to nerve root irritation |
| 4.25: Medial Collateral Ligament Injuries | **Pellegrini-Stieda sign**—avulsion fracture to superior border of medial femoral condyle |
| 4.26: Meniscal Injury | **Apley's grind test**—patient prone, knee flexed to 90°, apply axial force to foot → rotate tibia internally and externally on stabilized femur, pain means + test |
| | **McMurray's test**—tibial torsion with knee flexed at 90°, grinding or snapping means + test |
| 4.30: Osteoarthritis | **Bouchard's nodes**—hard nodules at the proximal interphalangeal joint (PIP) |
| | **Heberden's nodes**—hard nodules at the distal interphalangeal joint (DIP) |
| 4.31: Paget's Disease | **frontal bossing**—bony overgrowth of the frontal bone |
| 4.32: Rheumatoid Arthritis | **Boutonniere deformity**—flexed PIP joint, extended DIP joint |
| | **Swan-Neck deformity**—extended PIP joint, flexed DIP joint |
| 4.35: Scoliosis | **Cobb method**—lines are drawn along endplates of the upper and lower vertebrae that are maximally tilted into the concavity of the curve; then a perpendicular line is drawn to each of the earlier lines; the angle of intersection is the Cobb angle |
| 4.40: Spondyloarthropathies | **enthesopathy**—inflammation of tendon and ligaments at their insertion to bone |
| | **keratoderma blennorrhagica**—hyperkeratotic skin lesions of the palms and soles and around the nails |

### Chapter 5: Eyes, Ears, Nose, and Throat

| | |
|---|---|
| 5.8: Epiglotittis | **"thumb sign"**—seen on lateral x-ray of the neck an enlarged epiglottis and distention of the hypopharynx |
| 5.13: Hearing Loss | **Rinne test**—tuning fork placed alternately on mastoid bone and in front of ear canal tests conductive loss (bone conduction > air conduction) and sensorineural loss (air conduction > bone conduction) |
| | **Weber test**—tuning fork placed on forehead or front teeth tests conductive loss (sound louder in poorer-hearing ear) and sensorineural loss (sound radiates to better side) |
| 5.15: Macular Degeneration | **drusen**—variably sized yellowish, round spots deep to the retina and scattered throughout the macula and posterior pole |

### Chapter 6: Reproductive System

| | |
|---|---|
| 6.15: Newborn Evaluation | **caput succedaneum**—an area of edema over the presenting scalp that extends across suture lines; also seen at areas of vacuum extractor application sites |
| | **cephalohematomas**—bleeding in the subperiosteal space of the skull bones; the margins are limited by the edges of the involved bone |
| | **erythema toxicum neonatorum**—benign rash presenting like flea bites, with raised center on an erythematous base that may progress to vesicles |
| | **vernix caseosa**—whitish, cheesy material that normally covers the body of the fetus |
| 6.23: Pregnancy, Normal Signs | **chloasma**—darkening of the skin over the forehead, bridge of nose, or cheekbones; occurs after 16 weeks, called the "mask of pregnancy" |
| | **linea nigra**—darkening of the skin in the areola, nipples, and lower midline of the abdomen from the umbilicus to the pubis |
| | **mastodynia**—breast tenderness, caused by hormonal responses of the mammary ducts and alveolar system, varies from tingling to pain |

| **Review Card Number/Title** | **Terminology Links** |
|---|---|
| | **Montgomery's tubercles**—enlargement of circumlacteal sebaceous glands of the areola due to hormonal stimulation; occurs at 6–8 weeks |
| | **secondary breasts**—occur along the nipple line; hypertrophy of axillary breast tissue may cause a symptomatic lump in the axilla |
| 6.24: Prenatal Care | **triple screen**—screening test for neural tube defects and chromosomal abnormalities; consists of AFP, hCG, and estriol |
| 6.27A: Sexually Transmitted Diseases | **tabes dorsalis**—degeneration of posterior columns of spinal cord, resulting in Argyll Robertson pupil (does not react to light but does accommodate) |
| 6.29: Uterine Bleeding, Dysfunctional | **amenorrhea**—no bleeding for 6+ months |
| | **menometrorrhagia**—prolonged and/or excessive bleeding at frequent irregular intervals |
| | **menorrhagia**—prolonged and/or excessive yet regular bleeding |
| | **metrorrhagia**—irregular and more frequent than normal bleeding, but with a regular amount of flow |
| | **polymenorrhea**—regular and more frequent than every 21 days |
| | **oligomenorrhea**—bleeding < every 35 days and at least once every 6 months; also describes lighter than normal flow |

### Chapter 7: Endocrine System

| | |
|---|---|
| 7.1: Acromegaly | **mollusca**—fleshy tumors |
| 7.7: Diabetes Mellitus | **Somogyi phenomenon**—rebound hyperglycemia following an episode of hypoglycemia due to counterregulatory hormone release |
| | **syndrome X**—gradual development of hyperinsulinemia and insulin resistance before the onset of overt diabetes |

### Chapter 8: Neurologic System

| | |
|---|---|
| 8.4: Cerebrovascular Accident | **transient ischemic attack (TIA)**—neurologic changes lasting less than 24 hr |
| 8.15: Meningitis, Bacterial | **Brudzinski's sign**—flexing neck of supine patient results in reflexive hip and knee flexion |
| | **Kernig's sign**—patient supine with hip and knee flexed to 90°; further extension of knee causes neck and hamstring pain |
| 8.18: Multiple Sclerosis | **Lhermitte's sign**—sensation of electricity down the back upon passive flexion of the neck |
| 8.19: Myasthenia Gravis | **anticholinergic challenge**—administration of edrophonium will improve neuromuscular function in patients with MG |

### Chapter 9: Psychiatry and Behavioral Science

| | |
|---|---|
| 9.2: Alcohol Withdrawal | **delirium tremens**—an acute organic psychosis that usually manifests within 24–72 hr after last drink; characterized by mental confusion, tremor, sensory hyperacuity, visual hallucinations (snakes, bugs), autonomic hyperactivity, diaphoresis, dehydration, electrolyte disturbances (hypokalemia, hypomagnesemia), seizures and cardiovascular abnormalities |
| 9.6: Cocaine Abuse | **bruxism**—grinding of the teeth |
| | **delusions of parasitosis**—delusions of being infested with parasites |

### Chapter 10: Genitourinary System

| | |
|---|---|
| 10.1: Atheroembolic Renal Disease | **livedo reticularis**—semipermanent bluish mottling of the skin of the legs and hands, aggravated by exposure to cold |
| 10.4: Epididymitis | **Prehn's sign**—↓ epididymis pain with gentle testicular elevation |
| 10.5: Glomerulonephritis | **uremia**—S/S: anorexia, N/V, weight loss, metabolic encephalopathy, pruritus, pericarditis, peripheral neuropathy, bleeding |

### Chapter 12: Hematologic System

| | |
|---|---|
| 12.15: Sickle Cell Disease | **dactylitis**—swelling of fingers |

| Review Card Number/Title | Terminology Links |
|---|---|
| **Chapter 13: Infectious Disease** | |
| 13.8: Lyme Disease | **acrodermatitis chronica atrophicans**—dermatitis of hands and feet that progresses slowly upward on the affected limbs |
| | **erythema migrans**—cutaneous annular lesion with clear center and reddish periphery |
| 13.9: Mononucleosis, Infectious | **Burkitt's lymphoma**—a highly undifferentiated lymphoblastic lymphoma that involves sites other than the lymph nodes |
| | **hypersplenism**—increased activity of the spleen, in which increased amounts of blood cells of all types are removed from the circulation |
| 13.11: Neonatal Sepsis | **buffy coat**—light stratum of a blood clot when the blood is centrifuged or allowed to stand in a test tube |
| | **omphalitis**—inflammation of the navel |
| 13.15: Scarlet Fever | **strawberry tongue**—tongue is coated with enlarged red papillae |
| **Chapter 14: Surgery** | |
| 14.2: Appendicitis, Acute | **obturator sign**—pain with passive internal rotation of flexed leg |
| | **psoas sign**—pain with passive extension of right leg |
| | **Rovsing's sign**—pain in RLQ, caused by palpation of LLQ |
| 14.5: Cholecystitis, Acute | **Murphy's sign**—pain upon palpation of the gallbladder while taking a deep breath |
| 14.9: Informed Consent | **proportionate treatment**—treatment that, in the patient's view, has at least a reasonable chance of providing benefits to the patient that outweigh the burdens attendant upon treatment |
| 14.10: Inguinal Hernia | **herniography**—x-rays taken after intraperitoneal injection of contrast medium |
| | **Hesselbach's triangle**—bounded by inguinal ligament, inferior epigastric vessels, and the lateral border of the rectus muscle |
| 14.12: Pancreatitis, Acute | **Cullen's sign**—periumbilical bruising |
| | **Grey-Turner's sign**—flank bruising |
| 14.17: Ruptured Spleen | **Kehr's sign**—pain referred to left shoulder or cervical region due to ruptured spleen |
| **Chapter 15: Pharmacology** | |
| 15.18B: Pituitary/Hypothalamic Hormones, Continued | **Creutzfeldt-Jakob disease**—a progressive, inevitably fatal, slow viral disease of the CNS, characterized by progressive dementia and myoclonic seizures; affects adults in midlife |
| 15.24: Neurogenic Agents | **livedo reticularis**—a vasculitis affecting the skin; leads to a lacy appearance of red-blue "fishnet" mottling seen also with renal disease |
| 15.27: Antidepressants | **hypertensive crisis**—precipitated by eating tyramine = rich foods (cheese, fermented beverages), or sympathomimetic drugs (ephedrine) |
| | **serotonin syndrome**—facial flushing, hyperthermia, tachycardia, severe muscle spasm, rhabdomyolysis, altered mental status |
| | **torsade de pointes**—very rapid ventricular tachycardia characterized by a gradually changing QRS complex on the ECG |

# INDEX

Abbokinase, (*See* Urokinase)
Abciximab, 228
Abnormal digestion, 54
Abrasions, eye, 87
Abruptio placentae, 98
Absence seizure, 139
Acarbose, 219
ACE inhibitors, 203, 217–218
Acebutolol, 206
Acetazolamide, 202
Acetylsalicylic acid (ASA), 213, 227–228
Achalasia, 40
 surgical perspective, 189
Acne vulgaris, 160
Acoustic neuroma, 83
Acrodermatitis chronica atrophicans, 247
Acromegaly, 116
Acute abdomen, 40
Acute lymphoblastic leukemia (ALL), 172
Acute myeloid leukemia (AML), 172
Acyclovir, 235
Addison's disease, 116
Adenomyosis, 98
Adenosine, 201
ADH (vasopressin), 216–217
Adhesive capsulitis, 60
Adjustment disorder, 142
Adrenal crisis, 117
Adrenal hyperplasia, congenital, 117
Adrenocorticosteroids, 217–218
Adult respiratory distress syndrome, 28
Advicor, (*See* Niacin)
Agrylin, (*See* Anagrelide)
Albuterol, 205
Alcohol withdrawal, 142
Alcoholic liver disease, 41
Aldosterone antagonists, 217–218
Alendronate, 221
Allergic rhinitis, 95
Alpha blockers, 207
Alprazolam, 225
Alteplase recombinant, 228
Altered mental status, geriatric, 143
Alzheimer's disease, 128
Amantadine, 222, 236
Amblyopia, 83
Amenorrhea, 246
Aminoglycosides, 232
Amiodarone, 201
Amitriptyline, 225
Amoxicillin, 230
Amphetamine, 205, 226
Ampicillin, 230
Amrinone, 202
Amyotrophic lateral sclerosis, 128
Anaerobic pneumonia, 35
Anagrelide, 229
Anal fissure, 41
AndroGel, (*See* Testosterone)
Androgen inhibitors, 217–218

Anemia
 aplastic, 168
 hemolytic, 168
 iron deficiency, 169
 megaloblastic, 169
 pernicious, 170
Anesthetics, neurogenic, 222
Angina pectoris, 2
Angiotensin converting enzyme (ACE) inhibitors, 203, 217–218
Angiotensin II receptor antagonists (ATRAs), 203
Ankle brachial index, 243
Ankle fracture, 60
Ankle sprain, 61
Ankylosing spondylitis, 61
Anorexia nervosa, 146
Antacids, 210–211
Anterior cruciate ligament injury, 62
Anthrax, 178
Antiarrhythmics, 201
Antiasthmatics, 209
Antibiotic(s)
 aminoglycoside, 232
 bacterial cell wall inhibitor, 230–231
 carbapenem, 231
 cephalosporin, 231
 chloramphenicol, 233
 dapsone, 235
 ethambutol, 234
 fluoroquinolone, 234
 folate antagonist, 232
 glycopeptide, 231
 isoniazid, 234
 lincosamide, 233
 macrolide, 233
 metronidazole, 234
 miscellaneous, 234–235
 monobactam, 231
 nucleic acid inhibitor, 234
 oxazolidinone, 233
 penicillin, 230
 protein synthesis inhibitor, 232–233
 pyrazinamide, 235
 rifamycin, 234
 streptogramin, 233
 sulfonamide, 232
 tetracycline, 232
 trimethoprim, 232
Anticholinergic challenge, 246
Anticoagulants, 227–228
Anticonstipation medications, 212
Antidepressants, 225
Antidiarrheals, 211
Antiemetics, 212
Antifungals, 237
Anti-inflammatory medications, 213
Antimalarials, 214
Antiparasitics, 238
Antipsychotics, 224
Antiseizure agents, 223

Antithyroid agents, 218
Anti-TNF (tumor necrosis factor), 214
Antivirals, 235–236
Aortic aneurysm, 3
Aortic regurgitation, 23
Aortic stenosis, 23
Apgar score, 105
Aphthous stomatitis, 84
Aplastic anemia, 168
Apley's grind test, 245
Appendicitis, acute, 189
Aredia, (*See* Pamidronate)
8-Arginine-vasopressin, 217
Arthritis
 psoriatic, 80
 reactive, 80
 rheumatoid, 76
 septic, 186
ASA (acetylsalicylic acid), 213, 227–228
Asbestos pneumoconioses, 28
Aspirin, 213, 227–228
Asthma, 29
Asthmatic bronchitis, 29
Atelectasis, 190
Atenolol, 206
Atheroembolic renal disease, 151
Atorvastatin, 220
ATRAs (angiotensin II receptor antagonists), 203
Atrial fibrillation, 14
Atrial flutter, 14
Atrial septal defect, 7
Atrioventricular (AV) heart blocks, 3
Atropine, 204, 212
Atypical pneumonia, 35
Autoimmune disorder medications, 214
Autonomic medications, 204
 cholinolytics, 204, 208
 cholinomimetics, 204
 sympatholytics, 204, 206–207
 sympathomimetics, 204, 205, 208
AV (atrioventricular) heart blocks, 3
AV node reentry tach, 14
Avascular necrosis, 62
Azithromycin, 233
Azoles, 237
Aztreonam, 231

Bacitracin, 231
Back pain, low, 71
Baclofen, 215
Bacterial endocarditis, 4
Bacterial meningitis, 135
Bacterial pneumonia, acute, 35
Bactrim, (*See* Trimethoprim/sulfamethoxazole)
Barbiturates, 225
Barlow test, 244
Barrett's esophagitis, 45
Basal cell carcinoma, 165
Beck's triad, 243
Beclomethasone, 209

Bell's palsy, 129
Benazepril, 203
Benign prostatic hypertrophy, 99
Benzocaine, 222
Benzodiazepines, 225
Benztropine/trihexyphenidyl, 204
Bereavement, acute, 143
Beta blockers, 201, 206
Betaxolol, 206
Bethanechol, 204
Biguanides, 219
Biliary cirrhosis, primary, 43
Binding resins, bile acid, 220
Bipolar disorder, 144
Bisacodyl, 212
Bismuth subsalicylate, 210–211
Bisoprolol, 206
Bisphosphonates, 221
Bladder carcinoma, 151
Blood transfusion, whole, 199
Blount's disease, 63
Body mass index (BMI), 55
Bone, metastasis to, 73
BOOP (bronchiolitis obliterans organizing
        pneumonia), 243
Bouchard's nodes, 245
Boutonniere deformity, 245
Bowel obstruction, 42
Bradydysrhythmias, 12
Bran, 212
Breast carcinoma, 99
Bronchiectasis, 30
Bronchiolitis, 30
Bronchiolitis obliterans organizing pneumonia
        (BOOP), 243
Bronchitis, acute, 31
Bronchitis, chronic, 31
Bronchodilators, 208
Bronchogenic carcinoma, 32
Brudzinski's sign, 246
Bruxism, 246
Buerger's disease, 5
Buffy coat, 247
Bulimia nervosa, 146
Bulk laxatives, 212
Bullous impetigo, 163
Bupivacaine, 222
Bupropion, 225
Burkitt's lymphoma, 247
Burns, 190
    eye, 88

Calcitonin, 221
Calcium carbonate, 211
Calcium channel blockers, 201, 203
Calcium supplements, 221
Candesartan, 203
Candidiasis
    cutaneous, 161
    oral, 92
Capital femoral epiphysis, slipped, 79
Captopril, 203
Caput medusa, 244
Caput succedaneum, 245
Carbamazepine, 223
Carbapenems, 231
Carbidopa-levodopa, 222
Carbonic anhydrase inhibitors, 202
Carbuncle, 162
Cardiac asthma, 29

Cardiogenic shock, 5
Cardiomyopathy, 6
Cardiovascular system medications, 200–207
Carpal tunnel syndrome, 63
Carvallo's sign, 243
Carvedilol, 206
Cascara, 212
Castor oil, 212
Cataracts, 84
Cefazolin, 231
Ceftriaxone, 231
Cefuroxime, 231
Celecoxib, 213
Cellulitis, 178
Central retinal artery occlusion, 85
Cephalohematomas, 245
Cephalosporins, 231
Cerebrovascular accident, 129
Cervical carcinoma, 100
Cervical carcinoma staging, 100
Cervicitis, 111
Chancroid, 111
Chloasma, 245
Chloramphenicol, 233
Chlordiazepoxide, 225
Chloroprocaine, 222
Chloroquine, 214
Chlorpromazine, 224
Cholangitis, primary sclerosing, 57
Cholecystitis, acute, 191
Cholesteatoma, 85
Cholestyramine, 220
Cholinolytics, 204, 208
Cholinomimetics, 204
Chronic obstructive pulmonary disease
        (COPD), type A, 33
Chronic obstructive pulmonary disease
        (COPD), type B, 31
Cidofovir, 235
Cimetidine, 211
Ciprofloxacin, 234
Cirrhosis, 42, 244
    primary biliary, 43
Clarithromycin, 233
Clindamycin, 233
Clonidine, 207
Clopidogrel, 227–228
Clubfoot deformity, 64
Cluster headache, 132
Coarctation of aorta, 7
Cobb method, 245
Cocaine, 205, 222, 226
Cocaine abuse, 144
Coffee cup test, 244
Colesevelam hydrochloride, 220
Colestipol, 220
Collagen vascular disorders, 160
Colles' fracture, 64
Colon carcinoma, 43
Conductive hearing loss, 90
Condyloma acuminatum, 111
Congenital adrenal hyperplasia, 117
Congenital heart defects, 7–9
    atrial septal defect, 7
    coarctation of aorta, 7
    patent ductus arteriosus, 8
    pulmonary stenosis, 8
    tetralogy of Fallot, 9
    ventricular septal defect, 9
Congestive heart failure, 10

Conjunctivitis, 86
Contraceptive methods, oral, 105
Cor pulmonale, 243
Coronary artery disease, 11
Corrigan's pulse, 243
Corticosteroids, 209, 213, 217–218
Coumadin, (See Warfarin)
Courvoisier's sign, 244
Cranial nerves, tests of, 130
Creutzfeldt-Jakob disease, 247
Crohn's disease, 44, 244
Cromolyn sodium, 209
Croup, 179
Cubital tunnel syndrome, 65
Cullen's sign, 247
Cuprimine, 214
Cushing's syndrome, 118
Cutaneous candidiasis, 161
Cutaneous fungal infections, 161
Cutaneous parasitic infections, 161
Cyclobenzaprine, 215
Cyclopentolate, 204
Cyproterone, 217–218
Cystic fibrosis, 32
Cystitis, 158

Dactylitis, 246
Dalfopristin, 233
Dantrolene (Dantrium), 215
Dapsone, 235
De Musset's sign, 243
de Quervain's tenosynovitis, 65
Death, impending, Kübler-Ross stages, 147
Deep venous thrombosis, 11
Delatestryl, (See Testosterone)
Delirium and dementia, comparison of, 130
Delirium tremens, 246
Delusional disorders, 145
Delusions of parasitosis, 246
Demeclocycline, 232
Dementia and delirium, comparison of, 130
Depakene, (See Valproic acid)
Depressants, 225
Depression, 145
Dermatitis, 162
Dermatophyte infections, 161
Desipramine, 225
Developmental dysplasia of hip, 66
Dexamethasone, 213
Diabetes insipidus, 118
Diabetes mellitus, 119
Diabetic ketoacidosis, 119
Diabetic nephropathy, 152
Diazepam, 215, 222, 225
Dicloxacillin, 230
Digoxin, 202
Diltiazem, 203
Diphenoxylate, and atropine, 211
Diphenhydramine, 212
Disseminated intravascular coagulation, 170
Diuretics, 202
Diverticular disease, 44
Dobutamine, 202, 205
Docusate, 212
Dopamine, 202, 205
Doxazocin, 207
Doxycycline, 232
Dressler's syndrome, 243
Drotrecogin alfa, 227–228
Drug-induced asthma, 29
Drugs of abuse, 226

Drusen, 245
Duckett-Jones diagnostic criteria, 22
Duke diagnostic criteria, 4
Dumping syndrome, 191
Duroziez's murmur, 243
Dysplasia of hip, developmental, 66
Dysrhythmias, 12–14
    bradydysrhythmias, 12
    tachydysrhythmias, 13–14

Eating disorders, 146
ECG essentials, 15
Echinocandins, 237
Ecstasy (MDMA), 226
Ectopic atrial tach, 14
Ectopic pregnancy, 101
Edrophonium, 204
Egophony, 243
Elavil, (See Amitriptyline)
Electrical alternans, 243
Electrolyte disorders, 192
Emphysema, 33
Enalapril, 203
Enbrel, (See Etanercept)
Encephalitis, 131
Endocarditis, bacterial, 4
Endocrine system medications, 215–221
Endometrial carcinoma, staging for, 113
Endometriosis, 101
Enterocolitis, pseudomembranous, 197
Enthesopathy, 245
Epicondylitis
    lateral, 66
    medial, 67
Epididymitis, 152
Epidural intracranial hemorrhage, 133
Epiglottitis, 33, 86
Epinephrine, 205, 208
Epistaxis, 87
Epogen, (See Erythropoietin)
Eptifibatide, 228
Erectile dysfunction, 102
Ergot derivatives, 207
Erosive gastritis, acute, 47
Erythema marginatum, 243
Erythema migrans, 247
Erythema toxicum neonatorum, 245
Erythromycin, 233
Erythropoietin, recombinant, 229
Eskalith, (See Lithium)
Esmolol, 206
Esomeprazole, 211
Esophageal carcinoma, 45
Esophageal varices, 45
Esophagitis, 46
Estrogens, 221
Etanercept, 214
Ethambutol, 234
Ewart's sign, 243
Exercise-induced asthma, 29
Eye trauma
    abrasions, 87
    burns, 88
    foreign bodies, 88
    lacerations, 89

Felon, 69
Fentanyl, 222
Fibroid, uterine, 114
Fibromyalgia, 67

Filgrastim, 229
Finasteride, 217–218
Finkelstein's test, 244
Flecainide, 201
Flexeril, (See Cyclobenzaprine)
Flexor tenosynovitis, hand, 69
5-Flucytosine (5FC), 237
Flumazenil, 225
Flunisolide, 209
Fluoroquinolones, 234
Fluoxetine, 225
Flutamide, 217–218
Fluticasone, 209
Folate antagonists, 238
Folliculitis, 162
Fontaine diagnostic classification, 21
Foreign bodies, eye, 88
Fosamax, (See Alendronate)
Foscarnet, 236
Fosinopril, 203
Froment's sign, 244
Frontal bossing, 245
Fungal infections, cutaneous, 161
Furosemide, 202
Furuncle, 162

Galeazzi's sign, 244
Ganglion cyst, 68
Ganciclovir, 235
Gastric carcinoma, 46
Gastritis, 47
Gastroesophageal reflux disease, 47
Gastrointestinal system medications, 210–212
Gatifloxacin, 234
Gemfibrozil, 220
Gentamicin, 232
Gestational diabetes, 119
Glaucoma
    acute angle closure, 89
    primary open angle, 90
Glimepiride, 219
Glipizide, 219
Glomerulonephritis, 153
Glyburide, 219
Glycerin suppositories, 212
Glycopeptide antibiotics, 231
GnRH (gonadotropin releasing hormone),
    216–217
Gold, 209
Gold salts, 214
Gonadorelin, 217
Gonorrhea, 111
Gout, 68
GP IIb/IIIa antagonists, 227–228
Grand mal seizure, 139
Granisetron, 212
Granuloma inguinale, 111
Graves' disease, 120
Grey-Turner's sign, 247
Griseofulvin, 237
Guanethidine, 207
Guillain-Barré syndrome, 131

H$_2$ blockers, 210–211
Hallucinogens, 226
Haloperidol, 224
Hand infections, 69
Headache, 132
Hearing loss, 90
Heart block (1, 2-I, 2-II, 3), 12

Heart failure, congestive, 10
Heart murmurs, 17–18
Heart sounds, 16
Heberden's nodes, 245
Hematologic system medications, 227–229
Hematopoietic agents, 229
Hematuria, 153
Hemochromatosis, 48
Hemolytic anemia, 168
Hemophilia, 171
Hemorrhoids, 193
Heparin, 227–228
Hepatitis, 244
    acute, 48
    chronic, 49
Hepatitis A, 49–50
Hepatitis AI, 49–50
Hepatitis B, 49–50
Hepatitis C, 49–50
Hepatitis D, 49–50
Hepatitis E, 49–50
Hepatocellular carcinoma, 50
Hernia, hiatal, 51
Hernia, inguinal, 194
Herniated nucleus pulposus, 70
Herniography, 247
Heroin, 226
Herpes simplex infection, 111
Hesselbach's triangle, 247
Hiatal hernia, 51
Hidradenitis suppurativa, 163
Hill's sign, 243
Hip dysplasia, developmental, 66
HIV (human immunodeficiency virus) infection,
    179
HMG-CoA reductase inhibitors, 220
Hodgkin's lymphoma, 171
Homans' sign, 242, 243
Hormone replacement therapy, 102
Human immunodeficiency virus (HIV) infection,
    179
Human recombinant growth hormone, 217
Huntington's chorea, 132
Hydatidiform mole, 103
Hydralazine, 203
Hydrocephalus, normal pressure, 133
Hydrochlorothiazide, 202
Hydrophilic colloids, 212
Hydroxychloroquine, 214
Hyperaldosteronism, 120
Hyperparathyroidism, 121
Hyperpituitarism, 121
Hypersplenism, 247
Hypertension, 16–17
Hypertensive crisis, 247
Hyperthyroidism, 122
Hypertrophic pyloric stenosis, 51
Hypoglycemic agents, 219
Hypopituitarism, 122
Hypothyroidism, 123

Ibuprofen, 213
Idiopathic thrombocytopenic purpura, 172
Idoxuridine, 236
Imipenem, 231
Immunization schedule
    adult, 180
    pediatric, 181
Imodium, (See Loperamide)
Impaired absorption, 54

Impetigo, bullous, 163
Impetigo vulgaris, 164
Incontinence, 154
Infectious disease medications, 230–238
Inflammatory bowel disease, 80
Infliximab, 214
Influenza, 181
Informed consent, 193
Inguinal hernia, 194
Inotropes, 202
Insulin
    NPH, 219
    regular, 219
Interferon, 236
Intermittent claudication, 243
Intracranial hemorrhage
    epidural, 133
    subarachnoid, 134
    subdural, 134
Intussusception, 52
Iodoquinol, 238
Ipratropium, 204
Ipratropium bromide, 208
Irbesartan, 203
Iron deficiency anemia, 169
Irritable bowel syndrome, 52
Isoniazid, 234
Isoproterenol, 205, 208
Isosorbide dinitrate, 203

Jacksonian seizure, 139
Janeway lesions, 242
Jaundice of infancy, 53

Kabikinase, (See Streptokinase)
Kanavel's signs, 245
Kaopectate, (See Bismuth subsalicylate)
Kehr's sign, 247
Keith-Wagner classification, retinal findings, 91
Keratoderma blennorrhagica, 245
Kernig's sign, 246
Ketamine, 222
Kidney stones, 154
Klinefelter's syndrome, 123
Kübler-Ross stages, of impending death, 147
Kussmaul's sign, 243

Labetalol, 206
Labyrinthitis, 96
Lacerations, eye, 89
Lachman's test, 244
Lactulose, 212
Lamivudine (3TC), 236
Lamotrigine (Lamictal), 223
Lansoprazole, 211
Laryngotracheobronchitis, 179
Laxatives, 212
Legg-Calvé-Perthes disease, 70
Lepirudin, 227–228
Leriche's syndrome, 243
Leukemia
    acute, 172
    chronic lymphocytic, 173
Leuprolide, 217
Levine's sign, 242
Levofloxacin, 234
Lhermitte's sign, 246
Lidocaine, 201, 222
Lincosamides, 233
Linea nigra, 245

Linezolid, 233
Lioresal, (See Baclofen)
Lipid agents, 220
Lisinopril, 203
Lithium, 224
Livedo reticularis, 246, 247
Liver abscess, 53
Lomotil, (See Diphenoxylate, and atropine)
Loop diuretics, 202
Loperamide, 211
Lopid, (See Gemfibrozil)
Lorazepam, 225
Losartan, 203
Lovastatin, 220
Low back pain, 71
Low molecular weight heparin (Lovenox),
    227–228
LSD (lysergic acid diethylamide), 226
Lyme disease, 182
Lymphogranuloma venereum, 111
Lymphoma
    Burkitt's, 247
    Hodgkin's, 171
    non-Hodgkin's, 174

Macrolides, 233
Macular degeneration, 91
Magnesium, 201
Magnesium citrate, 212
Magnesium hydroxide, 211, 212
Magnesium salts, 211
Maisonneuve's fracture, 244
Malabsorption syndromes, 54
Malignant hypertension, 17
Malignant melanoma, 165
Mallet finger, 72
Mallory-Weiss syndrome, 54
Mannitol, 202
MAOIs (monoamine oxidase inhibitors), 205,
    225
Marijuana, 226
Martel's sign, 244
Mastitis, 103
Mastodynia, 245
McMurray's test, 245
Medial collateral ligament injuries, 72
Megaloblastic anemia, 169
Meglitinide, 219
Ménière's syndrome, 96
Meningitis, bacterial, 135
Meningococcemia, 135
Meniscal injury, 73
Menometrorrhagia, 246
Menopause, 104
Menorrhagia, 246
Menstrual cycle phases, 104
Mental status changes, geriatric, 136
Meropenem, 231
Mescaline, 226
Metastases, to bone, 73
Metformin, 219
Methicillin, 230
Methotrexate, 209
Methyldopa, 207
Methylprednisolone, 213
Metoclopramide, 210–211, 212
Metoprolol, 206
Metronidazole, 234, 238
Metrorrhagia, 246
Metyrosine, 207

Miacalcin, (See Calcitonin)
Midazolam, 225
Migraine headache, 132
Milrinone, 202
Mineral oil, 212
Mineralocorticoid analogs, 217–218
Minoxidil, 203
Mitral regurgitation, 24
Mitral stenosis, 24
Mitral valve prolapse, 25
Mollusca, 246
Monoamine oxidase inhibitors (MAOIs), 205,
    225
Monobactams, 231
Mononucleosis, infectious, 182
Montgomery's tubercles, 246
Mood stabilizers, 224
Morton's neuroma, 74
Mucosal stimulants, 212
Müller's sign, 243
Multifocal atrial tach, 14
Multiple myeloma, 173
Multiple sclerosis, 136
Mumps, 183
Murmurs, 17–18
Murphy's sign, 247
Muscle relaxants, 215
Musculoskeletal medications, 213–215
Myocardial infarction, 18
Myocarditis, 19
Myasthenia gravis, 137

Naproxen, 213
Neomycin, 232
Neonatal sepsis, 183
Neostigmine/pyridostigmine-carbamate, 204
Nephrolithiasis, 154
Nephrotic syndrome, 155
Neupogen, (See Filgrastim)
Neural hearing loss, 90
Neurogenic agents, 222
Neurologic system medications, 222–223
Newborn evaluation, 105
Niacin, 220
Niclosamide, 238
Nitrates, 203
Nitroglycerin, 203
Nitroprusside, 203
Non-Hodgkin's lymphoma, 174
Nonsteroidal anti-inflammatory drugs (NSAIDs),
    213
Norepinephrine, 205
Norpramin, (See Desipramine)
Nucleic acid inhibitors, 234
Nursemaid's elbow, 74

Obesity, 55
Obstructive sleep apnea, 34
Obturator sign, 247
Occupational asthma, 29
Ofloxacin, 234
Olanzapine, 224
Oligomenorrhea, 246
Omeprazole, 211
Omphalitis, 247
Ondansetron, 212
Opiates, and opioids, 226
Optic neuritis, 92
Oral candidiasis, 92
Oral contraceptive methods, 105

Oral hypoglycemics, 219
Ortolani test, 244
Oseltamivir, 236
Osler's nodes, 242
Osmotic diuretics, 202
Osmotic laxatives, 212
Osteoarthritis, 75
Osteomyelitis, 184
Osteoporosis, 124
Osteoporosis agents, 221
Ostium primum defect, 7
Ostium secundum defect, 7
Otitis externa, 93
Otitis media, acute, 93
Ottawa ankle rules, 244
Ovarian cysts, and tumors, 106
Oxazolidinone, 233
Oxybutynin, 204
Oxytocin, 216–217

Paget's disease, 75
Pamidronate, 221
Pancreatic carcinoma, 55
Pancreatic pseudocyst, 194
Pancreatitis
    acute, 195, 244
    chronic, 56, 244
Panic disorders, 147
Pantoprazole, 211
Paralysis, 137
Paranoid disorders, 145
Parasitic infections, cutaneous, 161
Parkinsonian agents, 222
Parkinson's disease, 138
Parnate, (See Tranylcypromine)
Parotitis, epidemic, 183
Paroxetine (Paxil), 225
Partial seizure, 139
Patent ductus arteriosus, 8
PCP (phencyclidine), 226
Pediculosis (lice), 161
Pellegrini-Stieda sign, 245
Pelvic inflammatory disease, 106
Penciclovir, 235
Penicillamine, 214
Penicillins, 230
Pentamidine, 238
Pentobarbital, 225
Pentoxifylline, 214
Peptic ulcer disease, 56
Pepto-Bismol, (See Bismuth subsalicylate)
Pericardial disorders, 19
Pericarditis, 20
Peripheral neuropathies, 138
Peripheral vascular disease, 20
    Fontaine diagnostic classification of, 21
Perirectal abscess, 195
Peritonitis, 196
Peritonsillar abscess, 94
Pernicious anemia, 170
Pertussis, 184
Petit mal seizure, 139
Peyronie's disease, 155
Pharyngitis, streptococcal, 187
Phenobarbital, 225
Phenothiazines, 212
Phentolamine, 207
Phenylephrine, 205
Phenytoin (Phenytek), 223
Pheochromocytoma, 124
Physostigmine-carbamate, 204

Pilocarpine, 204
Pinworm infection, 185
Pioglitazone, 219
Pitocin, (See Oxytocin)
Pitressin tannate, in oil, 217
Pituitary/hypothalamic hormones, 216–217
Pivot shift test, 244
Placenta previa, 107
Plavix, (See Clopidogrel)
Pleurisy, 34
Pneumonia, 35
Pneumothorax, 36
Podagra, 244
Polycystic kidney disease, adult, 156
Polycystic ovarian syndrome, 107
Polycythemia vera, 174
Polyenes, 237
Polymenorrhea, 246
Portal hypertension, 17
Positional vertigo, 96
Postpartum hemorrhage, 108
Potassium-sparing diuretics, 202
Pravastatin, 220
Prazosin, 207
Precose, (See Acarbose)
Prednisone, 209, 213
Preeclampsia, 108
Pregnancy, normal signs, 109
Prehn's sign, 246
Premarin, (See Estrogens)
Prenatal care, 109
Preoperative evaluation, 196
Prinzmetal's angina, 2
Procainamide, 201
Propofol, 222
Proportionate treatment, 247
Propranolol, 201, 206
Prostate carcinoma, 110
Prostate enlargement, 99
Prostatitis, 110
Proton pump inhibitors, 210–211
Prozac, (See Fluoxetine)
Pseudoephedrine, 205
Pseudomembranous enterocolitis, 197
Psoas sign, 247
Psoriasis, 164
Psoriatic arthritis, 80
Psychiatric medications, 224–226
Psyllium seed, 212
Pulmonary embolism, 36
Pulmonary hypertension, 17
Pulmonary nodule, solitary, 38
Pulmonary stenosis, 8
Pulmonary system medications, 208–209
Pulmonary tuberculosis, 37
Pulsus bisferiens, 242
Pulsus paradoxus, 243
Pyelonephritis, 158
Pyrantel pamoate, 238
Pyrazinamide, 235

Quincke's pulse, 243
Quinine, 238
Quinine derivatives, 214
Quinupristin, 233

Radiculopathy, 245
Ramipril, 203
Ranitidine, 211
Reactive arthritis, 80
Recombinant erythropoietin, 229

Refludan, (See Lepirudin)
Reiter's syndrome, 80
Remicade, (See Infliximab)
Renal cell carcinoma, 156
Renal failure, acute and chronic, 157
ReoPro, (See Abciximab)
Repaglinide, 219
Respiratory distress syndrome, adult, 28
Retinal artery occlusion, central, 85
Retinal detachment, 94
Rheumatic heart disease, 21
    Duckett-Jones diagnostic criteria for, 22
Rheumatoid arthritis, 76
Rheumatoid arthritis diagnostic criteria, 76
Rhinitis, 95
Ribavirin, 236
Rifabutin, 234
Rifampin, 234
Rifamycins, 234
Rimantadine, 236
Rinne test, 245
Risperidone, 224
Rosiglitazone, 219
Rotator cuff diseases, 77
Roth's spots, 242
Rovsing's sign, 247
rT3, 218
Ruptured spleen, 197

Salmeterol, 208
Sandostatin, (See Somatostatin)
Sarcoidosis, 37
Scabies (Sarcoptes scabiei), 161
Scarlet fever, 185
Schizophrenia, 148
Schizotypal personality disorder, 148
Sclerosing cholangitis, primary, 57
Scoliosis, 77
Scopolamine, 204, 212
Scurvy, 57
Secobarbital, 225
Secondary breasts, 246
Segond fracture, 244
Seizure disorders, 139
Selective serotonin reuptake inhibitors (SSRIs), 225
Senna, 212
Sensory hearing loss, 90
Sepsis, 186
    neonatal, 183
Septic arthritis, 186
Serotonin syndrome, 247
Sertraline, 225
Sexually transmitted diseases, 111
Shock, cardiogenic, 5
Shoulder dislocation, anterior and posterior, 78
Sick sinus syndrome, 242
Sickle cell disease, 175
Signet ring bronchioles, 243
Simvastatin, 220
Sinemet, (See Carbidopa-levodopa)
Sinus bradycardia, 12
Sinus nodal dysfunction, 12
Sinus tach, 14
Sinus venosus defect, 7
Sinusitis, 95
Skin carcinoma, 165
Skip lesions, 244
Sleep apnea, obstructive, 34

Slipped capital femoral epiphysis, 79
Smallpox, 187
Sodium channel antagonists, 201
Solitary pulmonary nodule, 38
Somatostatin, 216–217
Somatotropin, 216–217
Somatrem, 217
Somogyi phenomenon, 246
Spinal stenosis, 79
Spironolactone, 202
Spleen, ruptured, 197
Spondyloarthropathies, 80
Squamous cell carcinoma, 165
SSRIs (selective serotonin reuptake inhibitors),
    225
Status epilepticus, 139
Stimulants, 226
Stokes-Adams attack, 242
Stool softeners, 212
Strawberry nevus, 165
Strawberry tongue, 247
Streptase, (*See* Streptokinase)
Streptococcal pharyngitis, 187
Streptogramins, 233
Streptokinase, 228
Streptomycin, 232
Striant mucoadhesive, (*See* Testosterone)
String sign, 244
Strokes, ischemic or hemorrhagic, 129
Subarachnoid intracranial hemorrhage, 134
Subdural intracranial hemorrhage, 134
Sucralfate, 210–211
Sudden cardiac death, 22
Suicide, 149
Sulfonamides, 232
Sulfonylureas, 219
Superior vena cava syndrome, 198, 242
Swan neck deformity, 245
Sydenham's chorea, 243
Sympatholytics (adrenolytics), 204, 206–207
Sympathomimetics (adrenomimetics), 204, 205,
    208
Syndrome of inappropriate ADH (SIADH), 125
Syndrome X, 246
Syntocinon, (*See* Oxytocin)
Syphilis, 111
Systemic lupus erythematosus, 80
    diagnostic criteria for, 81

T3, 218
T4, 218
Tabes dorsalis, 246
Tachydysrhythmias, 13–14
Tactile fremitus, 243
Talar tilt test, 244
Tegretol, (*See* Carbamazepine)

Temazepam, 225
Temporal arteritis, 140
Tension headache, 132
Terazosin, 207
Terbinafine, 237
Testicular carcinoma, 112
Testicular torsion, 198
Testosterone (Testim 1% Gel), 217–218
Tet spell, 242
Tetracyclines, 232
Tetralogy of Fallot, 9
Thalassemia, 175
Thalidomide (Thalomid), 214
Theophylline, 209
Thiamylal, 225
Thiazide, 202
Thiazolidinediones, 219
Thiopental, 222, 225
Thromboangiitis obliterans, 5
Thrombocytopenia, 176
Thrombolytics, 228
Thumb sign, 245
Thyroid carcinoma, 125
Thyroid hormones, 218
Thyroiditis, 126
Timolol, 206
Tirofiban, 228
Tobramycin, 232
Tolazoline, 207
Torsade de pointes, 242, 247
Toxic megacolon, 58
tPA, 228
Tram tracks, 243
Transfusion, whole blood, 199
Transient ischemic attack, 246
Tranylcypromine, 225
Traube's sign, 243
Trendelenburg gait, 244
Trental, (*See* Pentoxifylline)
Triad asthma, 29
Triamcinolone, 209
Triazolam, 225
Tricuspid regurgitation, 25
Tricuspid stenosis, 26
Tricyclic antidepressants, 225
Trigeminal neuralgia, 140
Trimethaphan, 204
Trimethoprim, 232
Trimethoprim/sulfamethoxazole, 232
Triple screen, 246
Trousseau's sign, 242
Tubular necrosis, acute, 158
Turner's syndrome, 126
Type A COPD, 33
Type B COPD, 31
Tyramine, 205

Ulcerative colitis, 58, 244
Unfractionated heparin, 227–228
Uremia, 246
Urethritis, 111
Urinary tract infection, 158
Urokinase, 228
Uterine bleeding, dysfunctional, 112
Uterine carcinoma, and staging, 113
Uterine leiomyoma (fibroid), 114

Vaginal bleeding, abnormal, 114
Vaginitis, 111
Valacyclovir, 235
Valium, (*See* Diazepam)
Valproic acid, 223, 224
Valsartan, 203
Valvular diseases
    aortic regurgitation, 23
    aortic stenosis, 23
    mitral regurgitation, 24
    mitral stenosis, 24
    mitral valve prolapse, 25
    tricuspid regurgitation, 25
    tricuspid stenosis, 26
Vancomycin, 231
Vascular disease, peripheral, 20, 21
Vasodilators, 203
Vasomotor rhinitis, 95
Vasopressin, 216–217
Ventricular septal defect, 9
Ventricular tach, 14
Verapamil, 201, 203
Vernix caseosa, 245
Verruca plana, 166
Verruca vulgaris, 166
Vertigo, 96
Virchow's triad, 242
Volkmann's ischemic contracture, 81
von Willebrand's disease, 176

Warfarin, 227–228
Warts, common and flat, 166
Weber test, 245
WelChol, (*See* Binding resins)
Wellbutrin, (*See* Bupropion)
Whole blood transfusion, 199
Wound infection, postoperative, 199

Xigris, (*See* Drotrecogin alfa)

Yeast infection
    cutaneous, 161
    oral, 92

Zanamivir, 236
Zoloft, (*See* Sertraline)